Adventist Heritage of Health, Hope, and Healing

By
William C. Andress, DrPH

TEACH Services, Inc.
Brushton, New York

2008 08 09 10 11 12 · 5 4 3 2 1

Copyright © 2008 TEACH Services, Inc.
ISBN-13: 978-1-57258-490-7
ISBN-10: 1-57258-490-4
Library of Congress Control Number: 2007930164

Scripture taken from the New King James Version. Copyright © 1982 by Thomas Nelson, Inc. Used by permission. All rights reserved.

Cover photo—Artist conception of the world famous Battle Creek Sanitarium circa 1930.

Published by

TEACH Services, Inc.
www.TEACHServices.com

Dedicated to
Mervyn G. Hardinge, MD, PhD, DrPH,
Founder and Dean Emeritus of Loma Linda University's School
of Public Health

And to the memory of
Hulda Crooks,
Affectionately known as "Grandma Whitney."

This book would never have been possible without their Godly
influence on me,
through their practice of Biblical principles
of healthful living.

ACKNOWLEDGMENTS

I am indebted to numerous friends and colleagues for their encouragement and suggestions in making this book a reality. In particular I want to thank Martin Knopper, Bruce and Jeanne Farrell, Julian Melgosa, and Bob Wick for their editorial critiques that led to a more readable manuscript. Arthur Mallon and Wesley Taylor were gracious enough to take time from their busy schedules to review the contents before final publication. I am also grateful to the numerous individuals at TEACH Services, Inc. who worked behind the scenes to put the manuscript into marketable form. Finally, I want to express appreciation to my wife, Mieko, and daughter, Keiko, for their support and encouragement during the weeks and months when attention to this volume took up so much of my spare time.

—William C. Andress

CONTENTS

FOREWORD

From the very beginning God has offered choices to humans — choices of life or death, choices of health or illness, choices of hope or despair. This book invites the reader to make good lifestyle choices in order to enjoy happiness today, and to be ready to enter the kingdom for eternity.

This book offers a new perspective on the historic health reform proposed by Seventh-day Adventists. There is enough evidence from the forefront of scientific research to prove that the early visions given to Ellen G. White contained enough counsel to prevent a great deal of heart disease, cancer, obesity, diabetes, and strokes — the main killers of humanity today. The question of whether or not the Adventist health message makes a difference in wellbeing and longevity has been answered fully. The main purpose of this book is to establish that, even though adherence to this message will add years to one's life and life to each year, the matter of choice in health carries eternal consequences.

Throughout a careful historical and biblical analysis, Dr. Andress takes the reader from Eden to Egypt, to Canaan, to the middle ages and on to the nineteenth, twentieth, and twenty-first centuries. Across time, God has made sure that people had sufficient light to preserve physical and mental health in order to be prepared for salvation. Providentially, God has sent health messages at crucial times to ensure that his children are fit to carry out His mission and to be ready to enter Canaan, not only the Canaan of old, but the heavenly Canaan. Ultimately, the choice of health over disease may make a difference for eternity.

Much of the early history and development of the Adventist health message is depicted here with interesting facts, anecdotes and lessons to be learned from pioneers and recent heroes in the realm of health. This is a clear strength of this book, as history is written in a very attractive way, always with spiritual applications of each event.

Adventist Heritage of Health, Hope, and Healing contains a great deal of personal and meaningful experiences from the author. By means of personal interactions and professional experiences, Dr. Andress presents his main points in a powerful manner for the reader to comprehend and remember the importance and transcendence of the principles of health presented by Seventh-day Adventists.

This is not only a book to state the strength of the true health message, but also a deeply spiritual book where multiple biblical examples are outlined to offer attractive lessons geared to personal development, physically, spiritually, mentally, and socially.

Dr. Andress has made a successful attempt to offer many examples from the Bible, history, public health data, and personal experience to establish the main thesis of his book: The Adventist health message, if well understood, transcends the physiological realm and it is a message of restoration and redemption. It is one of the greatest needs of Seventh-day Adventists today and it is a message that needs to be presented boldly to everyone. For when this message is followed to its ultimate consequences, it will restore God's image into mankind.

Julian Melgosa
Former President
Adventist International Institute of Advanced Studies
Silang, Cavite, PHILIPPINES

October 22, 2007

INTRODUCTION

Solomon, the wisest man who ever lived wrote, *"Of making many books there is no end."* Ecclesiastes 12:12. So why another book on Adventism; especially when there are other volumes that contain the historical information found within these pages? In **Adventist Heritage of Health, Hope, and Healing**, I have sought to tell the story from a perspective that differs from the others.

The year was 1997. I was director of Health Promotion and Wellness at the Hong Kong Adventist Hospital. You may recall that 1997 was a watershed year for Asia, especially Hong Kong. On July 1, the enclave reverted to Chinese rule after being under British control for a century. Nineteen ninety-seven is also remembered as the year an economic crisis spread from Thailand throughout most of Asia.

Sometime during that year I began to ask myself the question, "Why did God give the Seventh-day Adventist Church a health message?" After all, no other group of Christians places as strong an emphasis on healthful living as do Adventists. And what exactly is the health message that the church should be preaching?

For almost 50 years, researchers at Loma Linda University have studied the lifestyle of Adventists. Results indicate that Adventists live up to ten years longer than their counterparts. This data is highly significant and has been widely published in the scientific literature.

Is this then the reason for our health message? So that we can teach our friends and neighbors how to delay death for one more decade? I don't think so. For if it is, we are merely teaching others how to be healthier sinners; and for a longer period of time.

As I grappled with the above questions, I discovered that many Adventists, especially new converts, know virtually nothing of the miraculous stories associated with historical Adventism. Such ignorance is not new. In Ellen White's later years she recognized that Adventists were in danger of losing sight of their roots. Around the turn of the 20th century she wrote: *"The record of the experience through which the people of God passed in the early history of our work must be republished. Many of those who have since come into the truth are ignorant of the way in which the Lord wrought. The experience of William Miller and his associates, of Captain Joseph Bates, and of other pioneers in the Advent message should be kept before our people. Elder Loughborough's book should receive attention. Our leading men should see what can be done for the circulation of this book."* [Reference is here made to The Rise and Progress of Seventh-day Adventists, published in 1892 by J. N. Loughborough (revised in 1905 as The Great Second Advent Movement).][1]

I also observed that any discussion regarding the "health message" has a tendency to polarize God's people. At one extreme are those who claim that a vegetarian diet and other healthful practices have nothing to do with salvation; the implication being that in the day by day scheme of things, such issues are unimportant.

At the other extreme are those who teach a philosophy that a friend of mine calls, "salvation by diet." These are the church members you do not want to show up at Sabbath afternoon potlucks. No matter what the dish, they will find something wrong with it unless it is the bland bean casserole that they have brought. To make matters worse, they vocalize what is wrong with everything else. With religious zeal smacking of Pharisaism, they make it known that partaking of such abominable food is committing sin against the Holy Ghost.

I would suggest that both positions are contrary to Scripture and that the truth lies somewhere in the middle. The principles of healthful living as found in the Bible, science, and the Spirit of Prophecy — when properly understood and applied — produce individuals whose lives are in beautiful biological balance.

1   White, Ellen G: *The Publishing Ministry*, p. 30

In my quest for answers to the "Whys," I arrived at three conclusions.

1) At the time Ellen White received her first health visions, life expectancy at birth in the United States was only around 40 years. Adventism's infancy is littered with the obituaries of God-fearing men and women who never made it into middle age. Thus the "health message" was literally a life-saving message so that God's people could reduce the likelihood of an early grave.

2) God wants his people to be healthy, happy, and holy. He suffers when we suffer, especially when the suffering is unnecessary due to either an ignorant or intentional violation of the laws of our being. The "health message" then is designed to equip God's people to live virtually disease free.

3) There is a close connection between our physical habits and our spiritual growth. The two cannot really be separated for what affects one affects the other. Thus the third reason for the "health message" is to prepare God's people for translation.

Initially I put together a series of vesper talks covering the topic. Over the years I have had the opportunity to give these presentations in various locations. Inevitably people have asked if these presentations were available in writing. The answer was always, "No."

Finally about four years ago, after I returned to the United States and began teaching in the Health Sciences department at Oakland University, north of Detroit, Michigan, I started to write out the lectures in manuscript form. What I thought would be a relatively easy task became larger and more complicated. First there were historical gaps that needed to be filled. As research continued, more intriguing stories were uncovered. Now it became a question of what to include; and in how much detail.

Obviously some readers will wish that greater information had been provided; while others will feel I have been too verbose. I hope that such impressions will not detract from the overall message that I am trying to convey. The underlining theme of this book is that throughout history God has been preparing a people to live with Him for eternity, and the "health message" plays a significant role in that preparation process.

In attempting to show how God has led in Adventism's past, I have interwoven my own personal story. I have graduate degrees in Public Health with an emphasis in preventive care. Unfortunately this does not make me immune to temptation. I find that far too often I struggle to consistently practice what I intellectually know to be correct. I grew up in an Adventist home but healthful practices did not receive a major emphasis in my childhood. Due to exposure at an early age, my taste buds acquired a desire for "that which is not good." Pastries, donuts, cakes, and pies were a delectable though deleterious part of my diet in my developmental years. In my ignorance I couldn't figure out why I frequently had a running nose and sore throat.

Heart disease was prevalent in both of my ancestral family trees. On my father's side, my grandmother died of a stroke in middle age. Though my grandfather lived until his late eighties, the last seven or eight years of his life were spent bedridden. He suffered from high blood pressure, diabetes, and strokes. On my mother's side, my grandfather died at a fairly young age from arteriosclerosis. My grandmother died in her sixties, after suffering her fourth heart attack. Both of my parents, especially my father, were overweight. Between them they suffered from heart disease, hypertension, diabetes, and other ailments.

I now realize that environmental choices were as much of a factor as was the inheritance of the wrong genes. My family didn't have set times for sleeping, exercising, praying, or relaxing. Life just sort of happened. Fifty years later I continue to grapple with these health destroying patterns established in my childhood. Especially is there a tendency to slide backwards under periods of stress and duress.

I share my testimony in the hope that it might provide encouragement to others who are struggling along similar paths. Though I'm not the man I once was, neither am I yet the man God would have me to be. Without the changes God has wrought thus far in my life, there is a good chance that I would have already experienced a premature death. I thank God that he is not finished with me yet. Praise God that in Christ, it is possible to overcome every inherited and cultivated tendency to evil. Yes, victory is possible. .

Still, day by day, I must be vigilant, and so must you if you want total victory. As you read, have an attitude of, "Lord, what will you have me to do? Are there changes that need to take place in my life? Are there things that I need to give up or stop doing because they are destroying this beautiful body which you have provided for the indwelling of your Holy Spirit?"

Then by the grace of God determine to take those actions which will enable you to experience *a heritage of health, hope, and healing*. Indeed it is God's wish for you my friend, to *"Prosper in all things and be in health, just as your soul prospers."* III John 2.

CHAPTER 1

FORSAKING THE TREASURES OF EGYPT

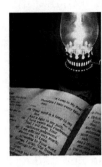

By faith Moses, when he became of age, refused to be called the son of Pharaoh's daughter;

Choosing rather to suffer affliction with the people of God, than to enjoy the passing pleasures of sin;

Esteeming the reproaches of Christ greater riches than the treasures in Egypt...

Hebrews 11:24–26

November 4, 1922 — Luxor, Egypt — For years, a team of archaeologists led by Howard Carter, had been digging in the rubble of The Valley of the Kings. On this date they uncovered what appeared to be the top of a stairway. As they dug deeper, unearthing first one step, then another, their leader could hardly contain his excitement. Could it be that at last he was on the verge of discovering the object of his dreams? Were his efforts over the last decade about to bring him to the apex of Egyptian glory?

The Valley of the Kings lies near present day Luxor. It became the final resting place of Egypt's greatest rulers from the beginning of the New Kingdom (1567 BC) onward. Down through the centuries Egypt's pharaohs and queens had been buried with incredible wealth in order that they might enjoy a reincarnated life in the Underworld. To the dismay of renown archaeologists, the significant tombs that had been discovered thus far had been plundered of their royal treasures.

Yet there remained one tomb that was thought to be still intact; that of the boy king, Tutankhamen. At one time believed to be the victim of an assassination plot,[1] King Tut had died at the age of eighteen and been hastily buried. But where?

No one was exactly sure. Pieces of funerary furniture, a blue cup bearing the name of Tutankhamen, and seal impressions of the king, had led Carter to believe that the crypt lay hidden in the Valley's ruins.

A deeply intense man, Carter was no amateur in the field. Years earlier he had played significant roles in the discovery of the tombs of Thutmosis IV, Queen Hatshepsut, and the intact tombs of Yuya and Thuya. Presumed to have been the grandparents of Tutankhamen, the mummies of Yuya and Thuya date back to the time of the Exodus.

Carter's interest in the tomb of Tutankhamen had actually begun in the early 1900's. Then World War I broke out and his excavations were put on hold. But after the war, his attempts at finding King Tut's grave were no more successful than before. Each dig ended in worthless mounds of shifting sand.

Now his sponsor and financial backer, Lord Carnarvon of England, was running out of patience. Already he had spent $2 million with only a few commonplace relics and piles of rubble to show for his efforts. He was ready to join the ranks of men like, Theodore Davis, the American archaeologist and financier who had gotten out of the business just eight years earlier. "The Valley is now exhausted," conceded Davis.[2] What he meant was that as far as he was concerned, there were no longer any worthwhile treasures buried there.

Lord Carnarvon also decided it was time to look for greener pastures. Or in this case, more golden opportunities. Carter had been given his fair chance. With nothing to show for his five years of investment, Lord Carnarvon was ready to withdraw his financial backing.

Like a snapping crocodile lurking on the banks of the Nile, Carter tenaciously pled his case. At last Carnarvon gave in, agreeing to fund the expedition for one more season. But only one more. For Carter it was either produce the goods or admit defeat.

Then came that memorable day — November 4, 1922. While digging beneath the workmen huts built during the construction of the tomb of Ramses VI, a water boy accidentally stumbled upon the stairway that must have sent blood pressures skyrocketing.

Two days later, excavation of the stairway was complete. Further progress was blocked by a massive doorway bearing royal seals. Carter felt certain he was on the threshold of something big. Yet his enthusiasm was tempered by evidence that the door had been breeched and then resealed. The rubble filled, 30-foot passageway on the opposite side gave further evidence that at sometime in the distant past the tomb had been entered and perhaps plundered.

After cabling Lord Carnarvon of his progress and potential discovery, Carter and his team could only wait and hope. At the end of the month, with Lord Carnarvon at his side, Carter stood in front of the sealed wooden doorway at the end of the passageway. No one knew what lay on the other side. Was it the wealth and fame that Carter had spent years looking for? Or was it nothing more than a dark, empty chamber; a sepulcher that long ago had been depleted of its treasures.

A hole was drilled in the upper left hand corner of the door. Holding up a candle to illuminate the inky darkness of the chamber, Carter peered in. Nothing was said. The silence was deafening.

Lord Carnarvon could no longer contain himself. Quivering and with bated breath he managed a whispered, "Can you see anything?"

Carter's response was simple, yet profound, "Yes, wonderful things!"

Later he would write in his diary, "At first I could see nothing...as my eyes grew accustomed to the gloom, details of the room within emerged slowly from the mist;

strange statues and animals and gold, everywhere the glint of gold."[3]

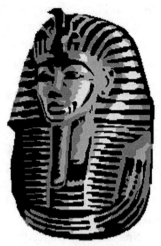

Here was immense wealth. Here were dazzling treasures from a bygone era. The glory of Egypt's past, untouched by human hands for 3,300 years, had been uncovered. Within days, news of the discovery of King Tut's almost intact tomb spread around the world. Carter himself would spend the next ten years meticulously cataloging the more than 5,000 items housed within the burial chambers; treasures that amounted to millions upon millions of dollars. Most spectacular of all was the 245 pound (110 kilogram) pure gold casket in which the boy king was laid to rest. Almost equally astounding was the gold burial mask which bore the royal likeness of the one awaiting his awakening in the hereafter.

The vast majority of artifacts can be seen today in the Cairo Museum in Egypt. However, the well preserved body of King Tutankhamen remains entombed where it was found in that sacred burial ground on the West Bank of the Nile, known as The Valley of the Kings.

Life in Ancient Egypt — The earliest Egyptian dynasties date back to shortly after the Flood. Initially the seat of government was centralized in lower Egypt, which geographically is situated at the northern part of the country or upper part of a map.[4] It was in lower Egypt, near present-day Cairo, where the early dynasties established themselves and where the great pyramids were built.

Economic life was based on agriculture, fishing, industry, and trade. Most Egyptians lived the simple lifestyle of a peasant. Housing consisted of a mud-brick hut, with a door and a few small windows. Wealthier nobles lived in either wooden, or higher quality brick houses.

Many of these houses had indoor toilets. Bathrooms contained a drain into a basin on the outside of the house. Sanitation was important and both the rich and the poor

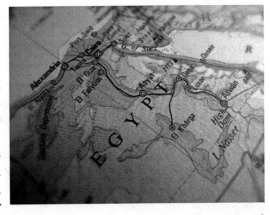

bathed frequently. Thus it would not have been unusual to find Pharaoh's daughter washing in the Nile River as she was at the time she discovered baby Moses floating in a reed basket among the bulrushes.

The ancient Egyptians were experts in astronomy, mathematics, and medicine. For example, they were the first civilization to adopt a solar calendar of 365 days and there is evidence of physicians performing a wide range of surgical procedures. Yet they are best known for their spectacular engineering feats, especially the building of the pyramids.

Engineering Feats — In the earlier dynasties, the pyramids were the burial tombs of the pharaohs. Most magnificent was the Great Pyramid of Cheops (Khufu) at Giza, one of the seven wonders of the ancient world. Actually this pyramid was just one in a series of three towering edifices that reached skyward above the barren desert floor.

The Greek historian, Herodotus, reported that it took 100,000 slaves working 20 years to build the 43 story colossal monument consisting of an estimated 2,300,000 limestone slabs. The workmanship was so precise that even today a knife blade cannot be placed between abutting blocks. How the builders were able to raise the facing stones, each of which weighed between 2.5 and 15 tons, to such great heights, remains a mystery. Yet recent findings documented in programs by the National Geographic Society provide a clue.[5]

In the early 1990's, archeologists digging on the Giza plateau made some startling discoveries that discounted previous theories. Within only a few hundred yards of the pyramids, a cemetery for workers was discovered. Further exploration led to the unearthing of a huge bakery containing large vats for mixing flour, numerous bread molds, and a brewery. To modern Egyptologists it was obvious that they were uncovering a city that had housed tens of thousands of workers who had been employed in the construction of the Pharaohs' tombs.

It is plausible that these workers could have been slaves. The book of Exodus begins with accounts of taskmasters forcing the Israelite slaves into stupendous building projects. *"And they built for Pharaoh treasure cities, Pithom and Raamses."* Exodus 1:11.

For years it was thought that the great limestone slabs were cut at quarries many miles away. They were then floated down the Nile on barges to the construction site. Again more recent discoveries provide an alternative explanation.

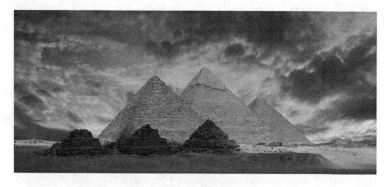

It seems that the Giza pyramids of the fourth dynasty kings, Khufu, Khafre, and Menkaure were built in the midst of an enormous limestone quarry. Thus the slabs only had to be transported a short distance. Evidence indicates that a ramp was built around each pyramid as the work progressed higher and higher. Teams of workers pulled large sleds bearing the limestone blocks up these ramps. Final placement and fitting of each block was done by skilled stone masons. With the placement of a capstone, each pyramid was completed. The ramp would then be broken down so that the rubble could be reused in other building projects.

Of the three Giza pyramids, the middle one belonged to King Khafre or Chephren, son of Khufu. This monolith originally stood 473 feet high. It actually appears to be taller than the Great Pyramid of his father, because it is built on higher ground. In front of the pyramid a causeway leads to a valley temple. Carved from a huge outcrop of limestone, the famous sphinx sits watching over this temple.

The Great Sphinx is 240 feet in length and believed to be a form of the sun god. In ancient days, it was an object of worship. Though still debated, most historians believe the face was carved after a likeness of King Chephren.

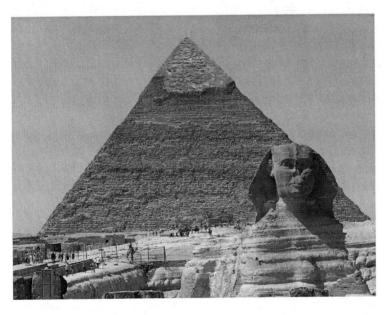

Because of the mysteries surrounding the pyramids, civilizations around the world maintained an interest in uncovering their hidden secrets. This was an undaunted task since the written Egyptian language of pictures known as hieroglyphics was virtually indecipherable. For centuries, Egypt's past remained shrouded in intrigue as inaccessible as the treasures plundered and carted away from her tombs.

Then in 1799, a rather large slab of basalt, known as the Rosetta Stone, was discovered by Napoleon's army. Carved in 196 BC, it was written in three languages; hieroglyphics, demotic or the common script of Egypt, and Greek, which since the time of Alexander the Great's conquest of Egypt had been the language of her rulers. For two decades after its discovery, unsuccessful attempts were made to decipher the hieroglyphics on the stone. The code was finally broken in 1822 by a Frenchman, Jean Francois Champollion. At last it was possible to make sense of the numerous descriptions found on tomb walls and inscribed on various artifacts. As a result interest in Egyptian antiquities was renewed.

Ancient Medicine — For the first time the ancient medical papyri could be translated. Nine of these medical texts have been discovered, and at least partially deciphered.[6] These writings shed enormous light on the diagnosis and treatment of disease in ancient Egypt.

The oldest of the texts is the Kahoun Payprus. Dating from around 1950 BC, many scholars believe it was actually copied from even older texts. Seventeen paragraphs address diseases of women. Other topics include assessment of sterility, pregnancy, and how to determine the sex of an unborn child. No surgery is prescribed; only drugs, fumigations, pastes, and vaginal applications are recommended.

The Edwin Smith Papyrus was a surgical textbook containing 48 cases, mostly head injuries. The cases were divided into descriptions of the malady, diagnosis, prognosis, and rules for treatment. For instance, a patient suffering from tetanus was to be placed in a sitting position with padded bricks under his armpits for support and a special instrument in his mouth for the administration of medications. In another case, instruction for measuring the pulse rate by means of a water clock was given. In examining the content of these writings, one historian concludes that they "reveal a knowledge of anatomy hitherto unbelievable."[7]

Discovered by George Ebers, the Ebers Papyrus is the largest and generally considered the most important medical papyrus. Dated shortly before the time of Moses, it is a medical textbook 108 pages long with over 800 prescriptions. At least a third of the drugs mentioned are still utilized by today's physicians.[8]

The first physician known by name was Imhotep, which means, "he who gives contentment." James Henry Breasted, a noted Egyptologist who translated the Edwin Smith Surgical Papyrus, believes that it was actually Imhotep who wrote that document.

Not only was Imhotep a medical doctor, he was also a statesman and builder. Sometime around

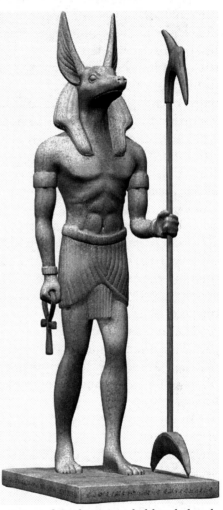

Statue of Anubis—A jackal-headed god in Egyptian mythology who lead the dead to judgment. In his hands are the staff of power and the "ankh," symbol of life.

2800 BC, as a tribute to his master, King Zoser, he built the world's oldest free standing structure, the step pyramid at Saqquara. Imhotep was held in such esteem by ancient Egyptians, that after his death he was deified.

In later dynasties it was the priests who largely filled the role of physician. Various paintings and carvings show the healers holding symbols of their importance in society. In the left hand is the staff of "power" while the right hand carries the cross shaped "*ankh*," a symbol of life from the sun. These symbols connected the physicians to the gods of healing and illustrate the high regard accorded to medical practice in ancient Egypt.

Interestingly, the *ankh*, that powerful symbol of life from the sun god, Ra, crept into the Catholic Church. The New Illustrated Great Controversy displays photographs of the inverted *ankh* in the shape of a cross rising out of a globe. In one photo, this pagan symbol adorns the papal tiara. The same figure of a cross atop a globe crowns a spire of St. Peter's Basilica in Rome.[10]

The Greek historian Herodutus, known as "the Father of History," noted that specialization was common among physicians. "Each physician treats a single disorder and no more."[11]

Some descriptions were quite specific. One doctor was called , "the guardian of the royal bowel movement."[12] Another ruler perhaps took this specialization a bit to extremes when he employed one ophthalmologist for his left eye and another specialist for the right eye.[13]

In the earlier dynasties, medical practices were rather advanced. There is evidence of knowledge regarding antiseptics, bandaging, ability to staunch the flow of blood, and how to set fractures and close wounds. Surgery was widely practiced. Archeological finds indicate a large array of surgical instruments including knives, drills, shears, saws, hooks, and pincers. A relief drawing on the door jamb of a tomb of a high ranking royal official shows two teenage youths being circumcised.[14] In both cases a crude flint knife is being used. The excruciating pain that must have been associated even with the simplest of operations makes one wonder whether or not such procedures were really worthwhile.

The extant papyri validate the large array of minerals, plants, and animals that were used in preparing medicines. Caravans traveled far and wide to collect plants that could be used in healing potions. Examples included aloe vera, frankincense, dill, caraway, garlic, mustard, onion, parsley, mint, and poppies from which morphine, codeine, and narcotine, were obtained. One remedy prescribed morphine for quieting a crying baby at night. Since morphine is a sedative, undoubtedly it worked well. And in some cases, perhaps too well.

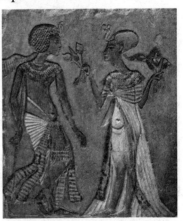

Another commonly used drug was mandrake. Primarily it was employed as a sedative in operations. But it was also believed to be an aphrodisiac and to increase fertility. A relief carving from the 18th dynasty depicts Queen Nefertiti offering mandrakes to her husband, Amenophis IV.

In Genesis 30:14–17, this belief in enhanced sexuality is illustrated within the story of Reuben preparing mandrakes for his

Relief drawing of Queen Nefertiti offering mandrakes to her husband

mother, Leah. *"Reuben went in the days of wheat harvest, and found mandrakes in the field, and brought them to his mother Leah. Then Rachel said to Leah, "Please give me some of your son's mandrakes."*

But she said to her, "Is it a small matter that you have taken away my husband? Would you take away my son's mandrakes also?" And Rachel said, "Therefore he will lie with you tonight for your son's mandrakes."

When Jacob came out of the field in the evening, Leah went out to meet him, and said, "You must come in to me;

*for I have surely hired you with my son's mandrakes. And
he lay with her that night.*

*And God listened to Leah, and she conceived and bore
Jacob a fifth son."*

Secrets of the Mummies — Nowhere though is Egyptian knowledge of medicine and human anatomy better
displayed than in the art of mummification. The Egyptian obsession with life after death led to the discovery of
a process that preserved the bodies of the deceased for
centuries.

Around the turn of the 20th century, an Englishman,
Armand Ruffer, began to study mummies. The techniques
he developed led to the science of paleopathology or
the "study of disease through the examination of fossil
forms." During the last one hundred years, more than
36,000 mummies have been dissected, x-rayed, and autopsied. Most of the mummies studied date from the later
18th to 20th dynasties. Since the editors of the <u>Seventh-day
Adventist Bible Commentary</u> believe that the Exodus occurred sometime during the 18th dynasty,[15] the study of
these mummies reveals much about health and disease
in Egypt at the time of Moses and the Exodus. The importance of this will be seen in the next chapter.

Mummification was an elaborate process. It was believed that sometime after death, Horus, the hawk god,
would return carrying the *ba* or spirit of the deceased.
Tomb paintings depict the *ba* hovering over a sarcophagus or coffin. The image of the deceased depicted on the
outer covering of the coffin was called the *ka*. If the *ba*
could recognize the *ka*, it would reenter the body and restore life. The whole purpose of mummification was to
preserve the body in such a way that it could be recognized by the *ba*. It was also the reason for placing the
deceased in an elaborate sarcophagus with a face mask
bearing a likeness to the corpse inside.

In the early years of mummification, the Egyptians
discovered that the internal organs did not preserve very
well because of their high water content. Thus, before

mummifying a body, the internal organs had to be removed. They were then placed in containers known as canopic jars. Each jar had a lid that bore a likeness to one of the four sons of Horus.

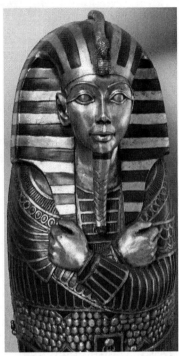

A replica of King Tut's face mask

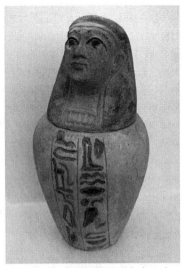

Canopic jar with man's head. Would have contained the stomach and large intestines.

Man's head = **MESTHA OR AMSET**	Jackal's head = **TUAMAUTEF OR ANUBIS**
Housed the stomach and large intestines	Lungs
Dog faced baboon's head = **HAPI**	Hawk's head = **QEBHSENNUF**
Contained the small intestines	Liver and gall bladder

For some reason, not much value was placed on the brain. By inserting a sharp instrument up the nostrils, the cerebral tissue was crudely removed bit by bit in mutilated pieces and cast aside. On the other hand, the one organ that embalmers did leave inside the body was the heart, since it was believed to contain the "seat of life."

Once the viscera were removed, the body cavities were filled with spices and the incision was sewn up. Then the body was placed in natrum (sodium carbonate) for 70 days. Subsequently the body was washed and wrapped from head to foot with bandages of fine linen, after which it was placed in a three-tiered casket made to conform to the shape of the human inside.

With Carter's discovery of King Tutankhamen in 1922, interest in Egyptology heightened. Though King Tut was a lesser king, Carter and his men were amazed at the millions of dollars worth of treasure with which he had been buried, some 5,398 items in all, including more than 200 articles of jewelry.[16]

For believers in the Biblical account of the Exodus, primary interest in Egypt revolves around events that antedated the reign of Tutankhamen by about 100 years. About that time, one of Egypt's most powerful female rulers sat on the throne. Her name — Hatshepsut. If, as many scholars believe, Queen Hatshepsut was the princess who rescued Moses as a babe out of the bulrushes, then she would have been his foster mother. And had Moses become Pharoah of Egypt, his reign would have taken place less than 100 years before that of Tutankhamen's. King Tut's tomb thus gives an enlightened glimpse into what Moses forsook by *"refusing to be called the son of Pharaoh's daughter;...and esteeming the reproach of Christ greater riches than the treasures of Egypt."* Hebrews 11:24, 26.

Had Moses made a different choice, perhaps it would have been his burial crypt that Carter would have discovered instead of King Tut's. Had Moses placed power, prestige, and position over a choice to serve God, perhaps today his name would be equated with the immense wealth of ancient Egypt. Perhaps tourists from around the world would be flocking to the Cairo museum to see the mummified remains of Moses, laying right there beside Egypt's noted icons; Ramses II, Amenhophis, and Merneptah.

But instead of inheriting the throne of the most powerful nation on earth, Moses cast his lot with a griping, complaining, rebellious group of slaves. He then suffered with them for forty years in a harsh wilderness. Finally the long trek of his life ended on the

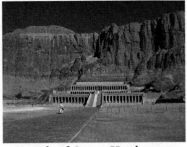

Temple of Queen Hatshepsut

banks of the Jordan River. On the other side lay Canaan, the Promised Land, flowing with milk and honey.

It was a land for which Moses had forsaken all the gold and silver of Egypt. Yet he would not spend a single day of his life there. After all he had left behind in Egypt; after all he had put up with in the desert; he fell short of his lifetime goal. Filled with sadness and disappointment, he trudged alone up the rocky slopes of Mount Nebo. From near its crest he peered across the Jordan into that glorious land that was not his to enjoy. While gazing with yearning desire, he reflected on the sin, so near the end of the journey, that cost him so dearly. And then, after receiving a vision of the future,[17] he lay down and died. Angels came and buried him in an unmarked tomb guaranteeing that its location would forever be hidden from the pick axes of tomb robbers, or the shovels of archeologists in later centuries.

In many ways, the life of Moses looks like it was wasted. After being groomed to become Pharaoh of the mightiest and wealthiest nation on earth, Moses threw it all away when in a fit of anger he murdered an Egyptian who was brutally beating a fellow Israelite. In fleeing the consequences of that impulsive act, he spent the next 40 years tending sheep. What a contrast! What a change — from powerful potentate to humble herder.

But during those forty years Moses learned patience, humility, trust, and complete dependence upon the God of the universe. Finally the day came when God could say, "Now, I can use this man to do great things for me."

You see, God doesn't call those who are great. Rather, those whom He calls, He makes great. And God called Moses, the tender of sheep, to shepherd His people while delivering them from the oppression of Egyptian bondage. Standing there alone on Mt. Nebo, Moses now reflected back on the miraculous crossing of the Red Sea, his ascent of Mt. Sinai to receive the Decalogue from the very hand of God Himself, the building the sanctuary, winning battles, and defeating God's enemies. Yet despite those triumphs, he now stood on the wrong side of the Jordan River, the side opposite his targeted destination.

Had it been worth the struggle? Was the price he paid to forsake the treasures and pleasures of Egypt too much? Surely it had cost him an earthly throne and an entry in the world's history books.

But because of that choice to surrender all to God, no matter what the cost in this life, the burial ground of Moses is as empty as any of the tombs in the Valley of the Kings. Yet unlike those graves and the burial chambers embedded deep inside the pyramids, Moses' grave was not plundered by some notorious gang of tomb robbers. No, instead the burial crypt of the prophet Moses was rent asunder by the King of the Universe. And today, instead of being a gazing stock wrapped in a natrium soaked shroud in the Cairo museum, Moses wears a robe of righteousness and walks streets of gold. Rather than the wrinkled leathery skin of a well-preserved corpse, Moses has the youthfulness of a new body; designed to never wear out. The mansion that he's inherited makes an Egyptian palace look like a hovel. And Moses even finally got his wish to set foot in the Promised Land when he was sent with Elijah to meet with Christ on the Mount of Transfiguration.

Before making that last solitary climb up Mt. Nebo, Moses stood before the congregation of Israel and challenged the camp with these words. *"I have set before you life and death, blessing and cursing: therefore* **choose life,** *that both you and your descendants may live:*

That you may love the Lord your God, and that you may obey His voice, and that you may cling to Him: for He is your life, and the length of your days." Deuteronomy 30:19, 20.

That same challenge still rings true. God's people have always been confronted with deciding between the glitter and glamour of the world (Egypt) or staking their lives on a "thus says the Lord," and walking by faith as did Moses. Dear friend, as you read the story of health and healing that is woven within the fabric of the history of the Seventh-day Adventist Church, remember it is a story about making choices. And as you read, be attuned to the voice of God speaking to you individually, challenging you to —

<u>Choose</u> the More Abundant Life!

CHAPTER 2

NONE OF THESE DISEASES

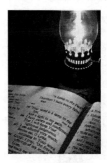

If you diligently heed the voice of the Lord your God, and do what is right in His sight, give ear to His commandments, and keep all His statutes, I will put none of the diseases upon you which I have brought on the Egyptians. For I am the Lord who heals you.

Exodus 15:26

June 1977 — Nagoya, JAPAN — The pain was excruciating. I could hardly breathe.

I had just finished a 12-hour work day during which the pains in my left breast had progressively worsened. By the time I finished teaching my last English as a Second Language class I was in misery.

In 1973, I went to Japan as a student missionary. It was the fulfillment of a lifelong dream. Growing up in an Adventist home I was surrounded with stories of missionaries from my earliest years. I especially enjoyed reading of the travels of David Livingston on the African continent, the Halliwells along the banks of the Amazon, and Eric B. Hare in Burma. My childhood excitement knew no ends when one Sabbath, "Dr. Rabbit," (as Elder Hare was affectionately known by the people of Burma) gave first hand accounts of <u>Clever Queen</u> in our church. I envisioned one day following in these missionaries' footsteps, and experiencing the rewards of a life built entirely on the ability of God to provide for my needs.

During my junior year at Columbia Union College, I roomed with Emmanuel Ascercion, the son of Filipino immigrants to the United States. One evening during study hall he approached me, "Bill, why don't we apply

18

to go as student missionaries to the Philippines next year. It will be a great experience for us. Plus I'll introduce you to all my relatives. We'll have a wonderful time."

Within days we secured a copy of the manual containing the calls for student missionaries. Much to our disappointment, there was only one opening for the Philippines; working in the radio station at Mountain View College, centrally located on Mindanao, the southernmost island of the Philippine archipelago.

Neither of us had the required qualifications for the position. Emmanuel decided that it was either the Philippines or nowhere. But by this time the enthusiasm of student missions had grabbed hold of me. Based on job descriptions and my interests, I filled out an application with my three top choices: 1) Teach English and Bible in Japan, 2) Teach Physical Education and Medical Cadet Corps in Ecuador, and 3) Assist in evangelism among the whites of Rhodesia (modern-day Zimbabwe).

Then I waited and prayed that I would be accepted. I didn't care where I was going, I just knew that here was my opportunity for mission service.

The General Conference assigned me to Osaka, Japan to teach English as a Second Language, and Bible classes for one year. That year in Japan was a watershed experience. Not only was it my first experience within a foreign culture, it was also a maturing experience as never before had I done my own cooking, cleaning, laundry, and shopping. I went to serve the country of Japan, and returned enamored with the country and its culture.

In August of 1975, I graduated with a Bachelor of Arts degree in theology. Since I did not have a sponsorship to the seminary at Andrews University, I returned to Japan to teach English as a Second Language. Eighteen months after my return, I married a girl I had given Bible studies to. We set up housekeeping in a small two room apartment, plus kitchenette and bath. Now just two months after our wedding, I was worried that these searing chest pains might portend an early widowhood for my wife, Mieko.

I figured I was too young to be having a heart attack. But what else could it be? I could hardly sleep as the pain continued through the night. In the morning Mieko made an appointment for me to see a physician who happened to be a member of our church.

It was a Friday when I visited him. After listening to my symptoms he proceeded to conduct a routine exam. Blood pressure — normal. Temperature — normal. Chest sounds — normal. As a precaution he decided to take several chest x-rays. Not having the equipment to develop them in his office, he told me he would bring them to church the next morning.

Sabbath morning I sought out Dr. Hayakawa. Not only did he have the news I was waiting for but he was one of the few church members in Nagoya whose spoken English was better than my fragmented Japanese. Holding the x-rays up to the light so that I could see them, he soberly said, "I want you in my office Monday morning to run some more tests. You have either pneumonia or tuberculosis."

Monday morning, in Dr. Hayakawa's office, I was administered the tuberculin skin test for tuberculosis. In less than 24-hours I knew what the diagnosis would be. The weal on my right forearm was almost two inches in diameter. Clearly I had a positive reaction to the test.

At the time, TB was one of the top five killers in Japan. Fortunately, before entering private practice, Dr. Hayakawa had been one of the leading physicians at a tuberculosis sanitorium and was an expert in the treatment of the disease. The first thing he did was confine me to bed rest for two weeks while he ran additional tests to determine how contagious I might be. During this time I was permitted to go out in public only long enough to visit his office every other day for intramuscular shots of streptomycin in my buttocks. I was also placed on a long term regimen of isoniazid (INH), a drug commonly used for the treatment of tuberculosis.

During that two-week confinement to "house arrest," I had plenty of time to think. "Why me, God?" I questioned. "I don't drink. I don't smoke. I'm even a vegetarian. Why should I get sick and not all those who are abusing their bodies?" Little did I know at the time that I too was abusing my body, albeit in different ways.

With a lot of time on my hands, I started listening to a series of tapes by Elder Glenn Coon on the ABC's of prayer. On one of the tapes he stated that the 28th chapter of Deuteronomy contained a whole list of curses that would befall God's people because even though they were "serving Him," they were not doing it out of the gladness of their hearts.

I pondered, "Hmnn. I wonder what's on that list."

Pulling my Bible off the shelf, I began reading Deuteronomy 28. The setting has Israel encamped in a valley between Mount Gerizim and Mount Ebal. Moses challenges the people to obey God and proceeds to dictate the blessings that would be theirs if they kept His commandments. Then he recites a litany of curses that would afflict them if they persistently disobeyed.

In the midst of the curses, Moses enumerates some of the diseases that would befall them. v. 22 – *"The Lord shall smite you with a consumption, and with a fever, and with an inflammation ..."*

I had no idea what "consumption" was. Flipping through my dictionary until I came to the word, I read, "The old term for tuberculosis."

Whoa! The words hit me like a ton of bricks. *"The Lord shall smite you with tuberculosis. . . ."*

I began to examine my life and asked God to show me what I needed to change. Mieko and I began to study The Ministry of Healing and Counsels on Diet and Foods, asking God to give us the courage and the power to make changes in our diet and lifestyle. I learned that even though I had been a vegetarian for more than 10 years, I had been a "junk food vegetarian." For years Sunday afternoons had been spent plopped in front of a TV watching the sporting events of the day while I consumed a large bag of potato chips and a couple of cans of soda pop. Nor was it a problem to eat three or four donuts in one setting.

In college, periodically I would go out with classmates to the local ice cream parlor to enjoy a pig's dinner. That was where we would gorge ourselves on all the ice cream we could for a single flat price.

I wondered why I was always sick with colds or the flu. Early on in my marriage, Mieko called me "Rudolph," after Rudolph, the red-nosed reindeer, because my nose was always red from blowing and wiping it. Having as many as five or six colds a year was not uncommon. And the worst thing about it was that I thought that this was normal. I believed I had inherited a weak constitution and there was nothing I could do about it.

My sleep patterns were erratic. Over the previous months I had been working 50–60 hour weeks as well as planning a wedding and looking for a new apartment. Mentally I was exhausted and often would engage in un-realistic negative thought patterns. And yet I thought that because I didn't smoke, drink alcohol, use drugs, or eat meat, I was following the health reform message.

As Mieko and I learned about healthful living, we be-gan to make some lifestyle changes; not all at once, but step by step. For example, refined sugars were largely eliminated from our diet. We started eating a greater abundance of fruits and vegetables. We got a juicer and began flooding our bodies with concentrated nutrients, extracted from the foods God prescribed in the begin-ning. Over time, high fat and cholesterol dairy products and eggs were virtually done away with. On doctor's orders my working time was reduced to twenty hours a week. This enabled me to start getting proper rest. I be-gan spending more time in the sunlight. I started drink-ing more water. As my strength returned, daily exercise became routine. And I began to spend more time seeking God's will for my life.

At the time, it was common for TB patients to be on a minimum two-year regimen of medications. Six months into my recuperation, Dr. Hayakawa said, "You do not have to see me any more. Your chest X-rays are clear. You are cured."

Preparing for Health Ministry — I remember think-ing, "Wow, if by changing habits of life, God can speed up the healing process, then there must be hundreds and thousands of people all around me who are sick and don't need to be. I'd like to help them."

But what did I know about health and healing? My college major had been in theology; not biology, or chemistry, or anatomy and physiology. In fact, I had avoided science like the plague. My undergraduate program had stipulated that I take a minimum of 12 credit hours in the sciences. So that's what I did. I took the minimum. Not only did I take the bare minimum, I deliberately sought out what I perceived to be the easiest courses.

There were four credits in Introduction to Math. I got a "B" in the course which I thought wasn't too bad. That is, until I met Mieko. She had been a math major. When she saw my college text she laughed and told me it contained the depth of mathematical concepts that she had studied in her freshman year of high school. Now that made me feel really great. But that's the way wives are. Somehow they have the ability to deflate the macho male ego and help us to get a more realistic grasp of life.

Another four credit hours were taken in Field Natural History. Here was a science course that I was able to get real excited about. The labs consisted of visiting coastal regions along the Atlantic seaboard to observe bird migrations, trips to the national arboretum to learn of the different flora and fauna, and jaunts to the national zoo to study mammalian species. Since I was fairly good at memorization and the course entailed mastering a lot of factual details, I managed to get an "A."

The third course selection, Introduction to Physics, was based on the input of Jeff, a friend who assured me that it would "be a breeze." The only problem was that Jeff was a physics major. Not only that, but he was somewhat of a prodigy. When only seventeen, he patented an eyepiece for a telescope. By the time he finished college he had even designed and built his own telescope. Of course an Intro to Physics course would have been easy for him!

But it wasn't for me. And since it was Jeff who had gotten me into the mess, I figured it was his duty to extricate me. I would go down to his room during study hall pleading for help in understanding the laws of physics and their applications. Jeff would spend 30 minutes cracking jokes, which did little more than irritate me. Finally he would look at the problems I was grappling with and within moments have them solved. Only problem was I still had no idea how to do them or what steps he took. Somehow I did manage to get through the course with a "B" and the conviction that the "sciences" were beyond my comprehension. I would stick with a less threatening subject like theology; or trying to explain who God is. So much for my naivety.

Due to my limited science background, when I returned to the United States, I initially spent a year studying natural healings at Wildwood Institute in the northwest corner of Georgia. During this time I became intrigued with the inner workings of the human body. With the completion of some additional work in Microbiology and Chemistry, in 1979 I was able to matriculate in the School of Public Health at Loma Linda University to study Public Health Education.

Sitting spellbound in Dr. Reuben Hubbard's, Historical Perspectives of Religion and Health class, I began to realize that the Bible was not a book just outlining the plan of salvation. I now saw that it was also God's instruction manual on how to enjoy a "more abundant life," in the present. In III John 2 it is written, *"Beloved, I wish above all things that you may prosper and **be in health,** even as your soul prospers."* And in John 10:10, Jesus himself said, *"I am come that they might have life and that they might have it more abundantly."*

Dr. Hubbard's profound knowledge of archaeology and ancient Egypt sparked my interest in the subject. One day he had us open our Bibles to Exodus 15:26. This passage contains the preamble to what is known as the Mosaic Health Code. These are the first recorded words spoken by God following Israel's crossing of the Red Sea. *"If you diligently heed the voice of the LORD your God, and do what is right in His sight, give ear to His command-*

*ments, and keep all His statues, **I will put none of the diseases on you,** which I have brought on the Egyptians. For I am the LORD that heals you."*

The Diseases of Egypt — After reading the above passage, Dr. Hubbard raised the question, "Wouldn't it be nice to know exactly what those diseases were? If God said that His people could live virtually disease free by following his commandments and statues, wouldn't it be beneficial to know just which illnesses He had in mind?"

Fortunately, the autopsied mummies, the medical papyri, the tomb paintings and other archeological findings from the era, provide a fairly clear answer to that question. There is reasonable evidence that smallpox, rickets, malaria, tetanus, tuberculosis, polio, goiter, worms and other parasitical diseases, pneumonia, and gonorrhea were commonplace. With the exception of smallpox, which was last seen in Somalia in 1977, these are the same type of infectious and deficiency diseases that are endemic in third-world countries today.

But it wasn't just the communicable diseases that were problematic. The discoveries from the past also tell of an Egyptian society that suffered from modern diseases of affluence. Heart disease, cancer, cirrhosis, gall stones, kidney stones, arthritis, osteoporosis, diabetes, constipation, anemia, dental decay, headaches, and gout, all wreaked devastation upon thousands.

The European historian, Jorgen Thorwald, stipulates that the wealthier classes in particular were just as likely to suffer from heart disease and obesity as is modern man. *"The mummies of kings Ramses II, Merneptah, Ramses III, Amenhophis III, and a great many lesser Egyptians, from the earliest to the latest periods of Egyptian history, revealed types of arterial diseases in no way differing from modern examples."*[1]

Two pages later he writes, *"Inspection of the skin, and especially the folds of skin, in the mummies of kings such as Thutmoses II, Ramses III, and Amenhophis III showed that they had been extremely fat."*[2]

Blindness was widespread. A major contributing factor was the epidemic of gonorrhea that existed largely due to the practice of temple prostitution. Today it is known that unless prophylactic measures are taken immediately after birth, gonorrhea can cause blindness as it is easily spread to the mucus membranes of a newborn's eyes when it passes through the birth canal of an infected woman.

Acts 7:22 states that Moses *"was learned in all the wisdom of the Egyptians."* This means that while being groomed to become Pharaoh, Moses would have studied all the Egyptian religious rites. He would have been immersed in the occult practices contained in The Book of the Dead. Since the Pharaohs were connected to the priests and it was the priests who were the physicians, it is safe to assume that Moses would have been educated in the medical papyri. He would have studied the Kahoun Papyrus, the oldest of the medical documents. He would have been familiar with the surgical procedures outlined in the Edwin Smith Payrus. Certainly the Ebers Papyrus, the medical textbook of the day, would have been perused. And Moses would have been familiar with the extant *Medica Materiale* on treating numerous diseases.

The Mosaic Health Code — With all his learning, it is surprising then that nowhere in the books of Exodus, Leviticus, Numbers, and Deuteronomy is instruction given on the diagnosis and treatment of disease. Perhaps his knowledge of Egyptian medicine is part of what God wanted him to unlearn while herding sheep in the Midian desert. For even though the books of the Pentateuch contain nothing pertaining to the treatment of disease, they do give detailed counsel on how to prevent sickness and stay well.

Otto Bettmann, the medical historian and founder of the prestigious Bettmann Archives in New York City, declares that Israel could not have survived 40 years in the wilderness without the guidance of a public health leader of genius.[3] Another writer states that Leviticus contains the "world's first written hygienic code."

The instruction given in the Mosaic Health Code can be divided into six major components. Of foremost importance was cleanliness; both personal and environmental. In Leviticus alone, over 60 references are made to washing or bathing. For example, Leviticus 15:13 admonishes bathing one's body in running water: *"...he shall count for himself seven days for his cleansing, wash his clothes, and bathe his body in running water; then he shall be clean."*

In the event that contagious diseases broke out in the camp, the afflicted were to be quarantined outside the camp. Such a practice was carried into Jesus' day. Thus we find the lepers were considered anathema, prohibited from mingling with anyone except other lepers. Wherever they went they had to announce their infectious condition by proclaiming "Unclean! Unclean!"

Sexual purity was tantamount. Not only did the seventh commandment speak out against adultery but other passages, especially Leviticus 18, made it very clear that incestuous relations, prostitution, homosexuality, and bestiality were all contrary to God's plan to preserve and keep His people pure and whole; physically as well as spiritually. *"According to the doings of the land of Egypt, where you dwelt, you shall not do; and according to the doings of the land of Canaan, where I am bringing you, you shall not do; nor shall you walk in their ordinances.... Do not defile yourselves with any of these things; for by all these the nations are defiled, which I am casting out before you."* Leviticus 18:3, 24

Dietary restrictions insured that the Israelites would eat only those foods that were most conducive to health. In the wilderness wanderings that meant a steady diet of manna; "angel's food"[5] or "the bread of heaven."[6] Upon entering the land of Canaan the manna ceased. Then the Israelites feasted on the fruits of the land;[7] not the carcasses of dead animals.

Flesh foods had been a mainstay of the diet in Egypt. Both Exodus 16 and Numbers 11 recount how the Israelites lusted for the flesh and fish of Egypt. In response to such clamoring God gave permission (notice it was permission, not preference) to include certain animals in their diet. Leviticus 11 and Deuteronomy 14 give the specifics of what was considered to be clean and unclean. "Clean," four-legged beasts had to both chew the cud and have cloven feet. "Clean" fish had to have both scales and fins. Predatory birds, reptiles, and certain other specified creatures were forbidden.

As an additional condition, even those animals deemed to be "clean," could only be eaten if they were fat-free and had the blood removed; a process that made the end result so distasteful that a Jewish friend of mine told me that the noted rabbi Mamomides suggested that it was really God's purpose that Israel abstain entirely from flesh foods. *"This shall be a perpetual statute throughout your generations in all your dwellings: you shall eat neither fat nor blood."* Leviticus 3:17. And to make sure that there wasn't any doubt, God went on to say, *"Speak to the children of Israel, saying, You shall not eat any fat of ox, or sheep or goat."* Leviticus 7:23. Notice it is specifically the eating of the fat of clean animals that the Bible condemns in this passage.

EGYPTIAN DISEASES
(based on the study of 36,000 mummies)

- Arteriosclerosis
- Liver Cirrhosis
- Diabetes
- Headaches
- Kidney Stones
- Arthritis

- Constipation
- Venereal Diseases
- Heart Disease

- Cancer
- Osteoporosis
- Obesity
- Dental Caries

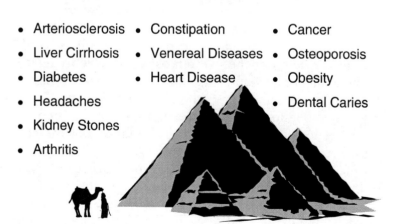

EXAMPLES FROM THE MOSAIC HEALTH CODE

PRINCIPLE	TEXT	DISEASES PREVENTED
Sexual Morality	Ex. 20:14. You shall not commit adultery. Lev. 18:22. You shall not lie with mankind as with womankind. Lev. 19:29. Do not prostitute your daughter.	STD's AIDS
Burial of Human Excreta	Deut. 23: 12, 13. When you ease yourself abroad, you shall dig... and cover that which comes from you.	GI diseases Typhoid Cholera Vector-borne diseases
Incineration of Waste	Lev. 4: 11, 12. Even the whole bullock shall he carry forth without the camp unto a clean place,... and burn him on the wood with fire.	Vector-borne diseases
Sterilization Procedures	Num. 31:21-24. ...Everything that may abide the fire, you shall make it go through the fire, and it shall be clean... and all that abides not the fire you shall make go through the water.	Various infections
Personal Hygiene	Lev. 15:13. He shall wash his clothes, and bathe his flesh in running water.	Communicable diseases
Quarantine of Communicable Diseases	Num. 5: 2, 3. Put out of the camp every leper every one who has an issue... without the camp shall you put them that they defile not their camps.	Infectious diseases, especially leprosy and skin diseases.
Tattooing Forbidden	Lev. 19: 28. You shall not make any cuttings in your flesh for the dead.	Hepatitis Tetanus

Prevention or Fungal Disease	Lev. 13:47-59. Care of clothing. Lev. 14:38-42. Treatment of houses.	Allergies Spore-borne disease
Exercise and Rest	Ex. 20: 8-11. Six days shall you labor but the seventh day is the Sabbath…In it you shall not work.	Stress related illness Diseases related to physical deterioration
Low Fat and Cholesterol Diet	Lev. 3:17. Eat neither fat nor blood. Lev. 7: 23-26. Eat no manner of fat of ox, or sheep, or goat.	Heart disease Cancer Diabetes

The last of the six broad categories in the Mosaic Health Code addresses the need to balance exercise and rest. This balance is beautifully depicted in the fourth commandment. Too often we emphasize the *"Remember the Sabbath day to keep it holy"* mandate, while forgetting the command also emphasizes working during the other six days of the week. Here is protection against man becoming indolent, while at the same time protecting against going to the opposite extreme and overworking, neglecting to take proper hours for rest, recreation, and recuperation. The commandment says to labor "six days;" not six days and nights. The fourth commandment is not just focused on a day of worship, though this is its primary intent. In its completeness it is designed to keep man in balance all seven days of the week. Bettmann recognized the therapeutic value of the Sabbath when he wrote, *"Most important of all, from a modern standpoint, the Jews set aside the Sabbath as a day of rest."*[8]

Stressed Out by Fast-Paced Lives — For six and a half years I served as Director of Health Promotion and Wellness at the Hong Kong Adventist Hospital. At that time Hong Kong had the reputation of being the "stress capital of the world." One news report stated that as many as

40% of the 6 million plus population suffered from stress related illnesses.

Hong Kong was also a very wealthy enclave still under British control. This was in the 1990's and despite its high cost of living, people came from around the world to try to make their fortune. Illustrative of the cost of living was the conversation I overheard while preparing to get my monetary affairs in order before moving abroad. The man conducting business in front of me mentioned to the clerk that his brother had recently accepted a transfer to Hong Kong because he would be getting a salary of $150,000 per year. When the clerk responded by saying that he would also jump at the opportunity for a salary like that, the man replied, "The only problem is that half of it is needed for housing."

I suppose that I too wouldn't mind spending $75,000 a year on housing if afterwards I had another $75,000 in discretionary funds left over. After moving to Hong Kong we learned that oftentimes $75,000 would only rent a high-rise apartment that was maybe 800–1000 square feet in size. We had friends who bought an apartment (Yes, in Hong Kong those who can afford to do so buy their apartment) that was about 900 square feet for the bargain price of about four million Hong Kong dollars (a little more than one half million US dollars.) Fortunately we were housed in the mission complex across from the hospital and didn't have to worry about paying such exorbitant rents.

Yes, in Hong Kong there is a lot of wealth but it comes at a high stress level price. More than one businessman was known to have spent his health trying to get wealth. Then while still at a relatively young age, he spent that wealth trying to regain his health in our hospital.

Such a lifestyle is insane. Yet in our fast-paced 21st century, more and more people are plummeting headlong down this pathway. When the prophet Daniel saw men "running to and fro," I wonder if he caught a glimpse of our society. Today's labor saving devices have only succeeded in allowing us to cram more and more activities into an already overly stressed condition. The research shows that modern man is too busy to find proper time for exercise, sleep, eating, quality family interaction, and most important of all — daily communion with God. The results of such a lifestyle are manifesting themselves in epidemics of coronary heart disease, cancer, strokes, lower respiratory diseases such as chronic bronchitis, emphysema, and asthma, diabetes, kidney diseases, Alzheimer's, and obesity.

Nor are these problems limited to the United States. While I was in Hong Kong a study showed that children in Hong Kong had the second highest cholesterol levels in the world, second only to Finland. Even in developing countries like the Philippines, coronary artery disease has become the number one killer. The island of Guam has one of the highest diabetes rates in the world. Japan, which boasts the highest life expectancy rates in the world, lists cancer, heart disease, and stroke as its major killers. And these diseases are striking at earlier and earlier ages.

God has a better plan for His children. He does not want you to be sick. He does not want you to suffer the ravages of a stress-filled society. So He has given instructions on how to relinquish the Egyptian lifestyle; for it is a lifestyle that produces untold stress followed by disease, distress, and premature death.

Results of Following God's Plan — What happened when the Israelites followed the statutes in the Mosaic Health Code? Psalms 105:37 says, *"He also brought them out with silver and gold, and **there was none feeble among His tribes.**"*

Then there are the specific records of men like Moses: *"Moses was one hundred and twenty years old when he died. His eyes were not dim nor his natural vigor diminished."* Deuteronomy 34:7 And Caleb: *Here I am this day, eighty-five years old. As yet I am as strong this day as on the day that Moses sent me; just as my strength was then, so now is my strength, for war, both for going out and coming in."* Joshua 14:10–12

Unfortunately, as we shall see in the closing chapters of this book, after reaching the promised land of Canaan, Israel failed to demonstrate the lifestyle that God desired for them. As a nation they rejected a vegetarian diet. Frequently they desecrated the fourth commandment. In sexual practices they became like the nations around them. As a consequence they never became the healthy, holy, happy people that God wanted them to be.

Far too often, the ability to replicate the physical feats of Moses and Caleb was diminished by the failure of the men and women of the Bible to adhere to God's statutes. Illustrative of this sad fact is the death of the high priest Eli. Remember, it was while Eli was officiating in the temple that Hannah dedicated her son, Samuel, to God's service.

While Samuel learned to love and appreciate the things of God, the same could not be said of Eli's sons. With them, Eli failed miserably as a parent. But he also failed miserably in following the Levitical teachings on health. Compare I Samuel 4:15 to the above account of Moses before his death. *"Eli was ninety-eight years old, and his eyes were so dim that he could not see."*

Continuing in verse 18: *"Then it happened, when he made mention of the ark of God, that Eli fell off the seat backward by the side of the gate; and his neck was broken, and he died: for the man was old and heavy."*

Eli had classic symptoms of diabetes. Diabetes is especially common in those who are overweight, and in the United States it is the number one cause of blindness among adults. Diabetics are also at greater risk of developing heart disease. Thus it is likely that upon hearing of the death of his sons in the battle with the Philistines, and receiving the news of the capture of the ark of the covenant, the stress was so great that Eli suffered a massive heart attack leading to his death.

Ellen White writes, *"Had they* (the Israelites) *been willing to deny appetite in obedience to His restrictions, feebleness and disease would have been unknown among them* (emphasis mine). *Their descendants would have possessed physical and mental strength. They would have had clear perceptions of duty, keen discrimination, and sound judgment. But they were unwilling to submit to God's requirements, and they failed to reach the standard He had set for them, and to receive the blessings that might have been theirs."*[9]

Nor were the Israelites the only ones to turn their backs on these teachings. Centuries later, during the Middle Ages, the Christian Church adopted and promoted practices profoundly in opposition to the Mosaic Health Code. As a result, for over a thousand years the Western world was ravaged by the most devastating plagues it has ever known.

CHAPTER 3

MEDICINE'S DEADLY DARK AGES

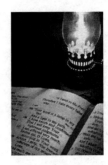

But you are forgers of lies,
You are all worthless physicians.

Job 13:4

December 29, 1170 — Canterbury, England — On this date, Thomas a' Becket, archbishop of Canterbury, was murdered while officiating at the cathedral altar. For many years he had been at odds with the ruler of England, King Henry II. Their heated arguments forced him to seek exile in France. While in France he excommunicated certain bishops for their support of the king. His refusal to absolve them threw Henry II into a rage.

A month before Christmas, Thomas returned to England to renew his duties at Canterbury. Other bishops saw this as the opportune payback time. In response to the king's fury, four knights tracked down the archbishop. With heinous brutality, his assassins vilified the sacredness of the cathedral as they hacked Thomas a' Becket to death . One blow split open his skull, spilling blood and brains upon the pavement in front of the altar. Following his death, the archbishop was canonized and his shrine became a mecca for pilgrims as highlighted in Chaucer's *Canterbury Tales*.

As monks prepared his body for burial they had to remove his priestly robes. In so doing they reported finding lice in his underwear "like boiling water." Repulsive as this sounds, it would not have been especially surprising for those living in the Middle or Dark Ages.

In the book of Leviticus, cleanliness is equated with holiness. *"That you may distinguish between holy and unholy, and between unclean and clean."* Leviticus 10:10. The health laws, including the dietary laws, were given within a context of holiness. After clarifying what animals are clean and may be eaten and which are unclean and to be avoided, God stipulates that the distinction is made because *"You shall be holy for I am holy."* Leviticus 11:44.

The message is clear. Israel is to follow a distinct lifestyle because she is a holy people. Physical cleanliness and spiritual wholeness are blended together. They cannot be separated. Yet this interconnection between the physical body and the spiritual life was largely lost sight of by both ancient Israel and the Christian Church in the Middle Ages.

Influence of Greek Thought on Western Medicine — In the wake of the Greek conquest of the Western world, Alexander the Great made Alexandria, Egypt his new imperial capital. Situated at the delta of the Nile, Alexandria was strategically located at the crossroads of Asia, Europe, and Africa. To its institutions came the best scientific and medical talent. Otto Bettmann points out that "the Alexandrian school of medicine influenced the training of doctors for centuries to come." In time it became particularly distinguished for its 700,000 scroll library.

Among the Greek physicians who engraved their mark on the annals of Western history was Pythagoras of Pythagorean Theory fame. He applied mathematical rules to the progression of diseases. Empedocles, one of his students, laid the foundation for the humoral system of medicine which dominated Western medical teachings for 2000 years. This concept taught that the four basic elements of the world — fire, earth, water, and air — had definite qualities of hot, cold, moist, and dry. These elements recurred in the body in the form of four fluids — blood, phlegm, black bile, and yellow bile. Disease resulted when these four elements or humours were out of balance. The work of the physician was to restore the balance of these humours in the body and thus bring about healing.

It was during the height of Greek power that Hippocrates, "the Father of Modern Medicine" exerted his influence. Today, almost two and a half millenniums later, graduating physicians still take the Hippocratic oath "to do thy patient no harm."

Among the ancient Greeks, except for Hippocrates, Aristotle probably had the greatest influence on medicine. Yet his teachings on "spontaneous generation," negatively impacted scientific advancement up to the 19th century. It wasn't until Louis Pasteur put forth his "germ theory" of disease in the 1860,s that Aristotle's fallacy of life springing spontaneously out of dung hills, was exposed in all its nonsense.

Greek mythology also played a critical role in the development of the healing arts. Aesculapius was the Greek god of healing. The Aesculapian staff consisting of a serpent entwined around a wooden walking stick is reminiscent of Moses holding up the brazen serpent in the desert. In worship to Aesculapius, temples sprang up all over Greece. Within their porticos the ill were given sedatives of hemlock and poppy seed while aromatic, perhaps narcotic smoke, drifted over them. The intent was to induce a hypnotic sleep. While in this trance, Aesculapius would appear and administer the remedy for each one's particular malady. "Cure" rates were enhanced by having patients undergo a preliminary screening process in which only those most likely to recover were considered eligible for admittance to the sick wards.

One prevailing teaching of the Greeks was the concept of dualism; a view that humans can be reduced to the two elements of matter and spirit. The body, being matter, was contaminated or evil. On the other hand, the spirit, which the Greeks taught was immortal, was good. Man's purpose in life was to develop the spirit to the highest level. Over time, this dual nature concept of man was adopted by the Christian church with dire consequences.

Ravages of the Middle Ages — During the medieval period the Roman Catholic Church reached its zenith. As predicted by Bible prophecy, its reign lasted for 1260 years, from the overthrow of pagan Rome until the Protestant Reformation eventually brought about its demise. Yet while the Church of Rome reveled in wealth and glory, the world around her entered a period of social, intellectual, physical and spiritual decline known as the Dark Ages. Akernecht in his <u>Brief History of Medicine</u> sees this period sandwiched largely between two great epidemics, the Plague of Justinian (542–543) and the Black Death which swept over Europe between 1348 and 1388.

The Black Death (bubonic plague) is regarded as the worst epidemic the world has ever known. Estimates of death range from one quarter to three-fourths of the population of Europe. In raw numbers, upwards of twenty-five million died. One writer says that the Black Death "threatened to exterminate the human race."

In some regions complete towns and villages were wiped out. Doctors were unable to do anything to stay the plague. How could they? Sickness was believed to be a curse either from God or the devil. Thus the "cure" lay in invoking the mercy of patron saints. Sacred relics were purchased in the hope that they would provide immunity. Treatments involved holy oils and magic potions. All were equally ineffective in stopping the devastation. Whenever someone did recover it was considered a miracle.

Nor was bubonic plague the only threat the medieval period had to contend with. Leprosy, smallpox, measles, tuberculosis, trachoma, syphilis, anthrax, cholera, malaria, typhus fever, dysentery, ergotism, diphtheria, influenza, scurvy, and diarrhea condemned hundreds of thousands to an early tomb. What caused such diseases to be so widespread and devastating?

Reuben Hubbard writes in his <u>Historical Perspectives of Religion and Health</u> that "The Biblical emphasis on cleanliness was lost in papal Christianity." He then declares that "the pagan belief of an immortal soul was adopted into church dogma" so that concepts of hygienic living were neglected and "living in filth became a sign of sanctity."

In other words, washing oneself meant undue attention to the body. Pagan Romans luxuriated in bathing. The ubiquitous bath houses flourished in an atmosphere that not only encouraged washing the body, but enticed open flaunting of sexual activity as well. For the Christian, the immorality could not be disassociated from the washing of the body. Furthermore, such undue attention to the physical body in and of itself, was deemed to be a sign of worldliness and living in extravagant ease.

Thus during the period of papal supremacy there was complete disregard for the principles of clean living spelled out in the Mosaic Health Code. The masses reeked of body odor. Clothes stank and were infected with vermin. The malodorous endemic led to the widespread proliferation of scented perfumes to mask body stench.

Towns and villages became virtual breeding grounds for disease and pestilence. The dirty, crowded conditions of the cities were accentuated by piles of garbage lining the streets. Cesspools overflowed with their effluence. No better environment could have been created for the proliferation of rats, flies, lice, mosquitoes, fleas and other carriers of disease.

Water pollution was another major source of sickness. Excrement from both man and beast seeped into the streams and rivers. Tanners contributed to the problem by washing their skins in the same waterways, while dyers poured their toxic residues into them. And all the while, in their ignorance, people procured their drinking water from these conduits of bacterial and chemical contamination.

Medical advancement during this period was stymied by three papal edicts. The first was issued in 1163 at the Council of Tours. The pronouncement, "the church does not shed blood,"[6] was followed half a century later with Pope Innocent III's proclamation of an anathema against surgery.[7] The combined result was to take away the surgical lancet from the physicians, who for the most part were clergymen, and put it into the unscrupulous hands of barbers and bathhouse attendants.

In 1219, at the Council of Rheims, the Church administered its second death knell when it forbad monks to even practice medicine.[8] The final blow was struck in 1300 when Pope Boniface VIII issued a decree against the dissection of dead bodies.[9] This effectually put an end to any study of anatomy and physiology and led to the stagnation of medical advances throughout Western Europe for several hundred years.

The one bright spot in the midst of this morass, was the founding of the first hospital in Salerno, Italy. It emerged around 900 in a salubrious climate off the coast of Italy. For the first time the term *physicus*, from which we get our word "physician," was used to refer to doctors.[10] An eclectic approach of rational interventions along with natural remedies was employed. Unfortunately its fame led to the promulgation of some fallacies that would be practiced for centuries.

Introduction of Bleeding As a Panacea for Disease — Remember the Greeks taught that an imbalance of the humours lead to illness. It was thought that the four humours (blood, phlegm, yellow bile, and black bile) were somehow intermingled or connected, possibly through tubes. Since blood was the fluid most readily available, it was believed that by removing any "excess blood" balance could be restored among the humours. Thus began the practice of bloodletting or bleeding. This practice became a panacea for treating almost every disease and dominated Western medical thought well into the nineteenth century.

As medicine sank deeper and deeper into superstition, astrological charts were prepared to guide the illiterate barbers in making their decisions regarding when and where to bleed the patient. In such a milieu of ignorance it is no wonder that the afflicted sought healing through exorcisms, incantations, prayers of penitence, and the invocation of patron saints. As Hubbard so aptly points out, *"While the Roman Church may have deliberately put to death thousands through the Inquisition, she inadvertently caused the death of thousands more through her stifling dogmas which fostered superstition, ignorance, and unhealthful practices."*[11]

The Roman Church's downfall began in 1517 with Martin Luther's nailing of the 95 theses to the church door in Wittenberg. The Protestant Reformation unleashed by that single act proved to be the salvation of the medieval world — spiritually, mentally, and physically — "for with the Reformation came a new emphasis upon scientific medicine and rational health practices."[12]

Still it would take more than 350 years before medicine achieved the rational reputation for which it is noted today. And the Seventh-day Adventist Church was destined to play a significant role in that transformation.

CHAPTER 4

DAYS OF BLOOD, DRUGS, AND TEARS

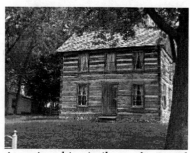

My people are destroyed for lack of knowledge.

Hosea 4:6

1851 — Somerville, Massachusetts — Joseph Bates had a dream. Now it wasn't unusual for the former sea captain to have dreams. Significant dreams. Dreams in which God led him directly to people who were ready to hear the gospel.[1]

One of his most amazing dreams was the one he had while heading west to hold evangelistic meetings in Indiana. On the way he stopped in Jackson, Michigan. There he dreamed of being on a steamship sailing to Battle Creek. Elder Bates had never heard of Battle Creek. But impressed that God was directing him, he booked passage on a train and headed for this small town 40 miles west of Jackson.

Arriving in the early morning, he had no idea where to go. He was in a strange environment and knew nobody in the area. Praying for God's guidance he went to the post office. There he asked for "the most honest man in town."

A rustic cabin similar to the David Hewitt home.

The postmaster directed Elder Bates to the rustic

42

cabin of David Hewitt on Van Buren St. in the west part of town. The Hewitts were just sitting down to breakfast when Bates knocked on the door. When Mr. Hewitt answered it, Joseph explained to him that he had some important Biblical news for "the most honest man in town," and had been directed to his home. David agreed to listen; after they first ate breakfast together.

With breakfast finished, the Hewitt family sat spellbound as Elder Bates unfurled his charts and explained the prophecies of Daniel 2, 7, and 8. All morning and afternoon the Bible study continued. By sundown, David and his family had accepted the seventh-day Sabbath and became the first converts to Adventism in Battle Creek.

Two years later, it was in the front room of the Hewitt's humble house where the Whites held their first meeting in Battle Creek. And a few years later it was David Hewitt who suggested that the rapidly growing group of Adventist believers be known by the name *Seventh-day Adventists*.

But back to the dream in Somerville. It happened on a Friday night. Elder Bates had been invited to hold evangelistic meetings at the home of an Advent believer in Somerville, a suburb of Boston. Bates had never been to this home before, but in the dream he saw in detail the room in which he was preaching. Every seat was occupied except one by the rear door. The congregation had just finished singing the second hymn when he stood up and began to read from Daniel 8:14, "*Unto two thousand and three hundred days, then shall the sanctuary be cleansed.*" At that very moment, a young girl walk in and took the one remaining seat. He dreamed that her name was Annie Smith.

Annie Rebekah Smith was the only daughter of Samuel and Rebekah Spalding Smith. Her brother, Uriah, is better known to most Adventists. For many years Elder Uriah Smith was the editor of the *Review and Herald*, and later wrote the exhaustive commentary Thoughts on Daniel and the Revelation.

In the religious fervor of the 1840's, Annie joined the Millerite movement. But like so many other Millerites, after the Great Disappointment of October 22, 1844, she lost interest in religion and the Biblical teachings on the second coming of Christ. Trained as a teacher, she was just getting established in her profession when she received a letter from her mother inviting her to attend meetings being held by Bates in a nearby town. She really wasn't too excited about attending, but in order to pacify her mother, she decided to go to the first meeting. Besides it was on a Saturday and she didn't have to work.

Like Elder Bates, she too had a dream about this event. In it she arrived late, sat near the back door, and heard a sermon on the 2300 days of Daniel 8:14. On the day of the actual meeting, she left her home in plenty of time but got lost on the way. Arriving late she slipped in the back where she took a seat near the door and saw the rest of her dream, and Elder Bates' dream, fulfilled in every detail. Conviction struck her heart.

Within three weeks she decided to join the emerging body of Sabbath keepers. Soon she employed her poetic skills in writing for the *Sabbath Review and Advent Herald*, the church's official paper. It wasn't long before her proofreading and copy editing talents promoted her to the position of assistant editor.

Three of her hymns, *"How Far From Home," "I Saw One Weary," and "Long Upon the Mountains,"* appear in the current Seventh-day Adventist Church Hymnal. Hymn number 441, *"I Saw One Weary,"* encapsulates the experience of three early Adventist pioneers, Joseph Bates, James White, and according to Annie's mother, Annie herself.

"I saw one weary, sad, and torn, With eager steps press on the way,
Who long the hallowed cross had borne, . . .
I asked what buoyed his spirits up, "Oh, this!" said he
— "The blessed hope."

It was Joseph Bates who always signed his letters with encouragement from Titus 2:13, *"Yours in the blessed hope."*

The second stanza highlights the struggles of James White.

"And one I saw, with sword and shield, Who boldly braved the world's cold frown,
And fought unyielding on the field, To win an everlasting crown.
Though worn with toil, oppressed by foes..."

The virtual leader of the early Advent church, Elder White faced poverty, fanaticism, and other hardships. Untiring in ceaseless efforts to advance the cause he so fervently believed in, he too remained firm in his hope of the second advent.

"And there was one who left behind the cherished friends of early years,
And honor, pleasure, wealth resigned, To tread the path bedewed with tears.
Through trials deep and conflicts sore, yet still a smile of joy he wore...."

For consistency, Annie maintained the masculine gender. Yet the words of the third stanza certainly describe Annie's personal experience of giving up friends, career, and financial gain in order to lend her talents to the remnant church.

For four years her work with the *Advent Review and Sabbath Herald* was greatly appreciated. In 1855, a collection of 25 of her hymns and numerous other poems, <u>Home Here, and Home in Heaven</u>, was published. The preface was written the night before she succumbed to the ravages of tuberculosis. Age — 27-years-old.

In the mid-1800's, early death was the rule rather than the exception. Oak Hill Cemetery, located in the midst of a tree-lined residential neighborhood south of

Battle Creek, is populated with tombstones telling the stories of lives far too often snuffed out in infancy, early childhood, the teens, and young adulthood. At the time the Adventist Church was going through its birthing pains, life expectancy in the United States was less than forty years. Sickness

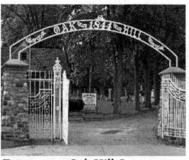

Entrance to Oak Hill Cemetery as it appears today. Notice the year in which it was founded.

and premature death were a standard part of life.

Mary Kellogg, the first wife of John Preston Kellogg, also died from consumption at an early age. Her death occurred shortly after the birth of her fifth child. J. N. Loughborough, an early Adventist minister, recalled how at the age of eight he witnessed his father, afflicted with typhoid fever, being denied any fresh air or cool water while being lovingly poisoned to death with drugs.

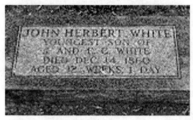

Nor were James and Ellen White spared. In 1860, their youngest son, Herbert, died just short of being three-months-old. Three years later, their eldest son Henry, passed away at the tender age of sixteen. Notice these passages from Ellen White's autobiography as she tells of the grief that beset her home.

"*When that tender branch was broken* (death of Herbert), *how our hearts did bleed... But oh, when our noble Henry died, at the age of sixteen ... ours was a lonely home... But God comforted us in our bereavements and we pressed*

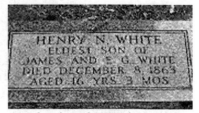

Herbert's and Henry's tombs in the White family plot at Oak Hill Cemetery *forward in the work He had given us, in bright hope of meeting our children who had been torn from us by death, in that world where sickness and death will never come."*[2]

A few pages earlier she had written of the premature demise of her brother. *"Soon after our family became settled in Rochester, we received a letter from my mother informing us of the dangerous illness of my brother Robert, who lived with my parents in Gorham, Maine. When the news of his sickness reached us, my sister Sarah decided to go immediately to Gorham.*

To all appearance my brother could live but a few days; yet contrary to the expectations of all, he lingered for six months, a great sufferer. My sister faithfully watched over him until the last. We had the privilege of visiting him before his death. It was an affecting meeting. He was much changed, yet his wasted features were lighted up with joy. Bright hope of the future constantly sustained him. We had seasons of prayer in his room, and Jesus seemed very near. We were obliged to separate from our dear brother, expecting never to meet him again this side of the resurrection of the just. Soon afterward my brother fell asleep in Jesus, in full hope of having a part in the first resurrection."[3]

In the same book Ellen tells of arranging for James' brother, Nathaniel, and his wife to come and live with them awhile as they both were invalids. *"As soon as we saw Nathaniel, we feared that consumption had marked him for the grave. ...*

May 6, 1853, we prepared Nathaniel's supper, but he soon said that he was faint, and did not know but that he was going to die. He sent for me, and as soon as I entered the room, I knew that he was dying, and said to him: "Nathaniel dear, trust in God. He loves you, and you love Him. Trust in Him as a child trusts in its parents. Don't be troubled. The Lord will not leave you." Said he, "Yes, yes." We prayed, and he responded, "Amen, praise the Lord!" He did not seem to suffer pain. He did not groan once, or struggle, or move a muscle of his face, but breathed shorter and shorter until he fell asleep, in the twenty- second year of his age."[4]

God wants His people to be happy. He wants them to be healthy. Above all, God wants a people that are holy. Jesus came to this earth to restore in man the image of God, "It was His mission to bring men complete restoration; He came to give them health, peace, and perfection of character."[5] But in the mid-1800's, God's people were anything but happy, healthy, and holy. More accurately they were sad, sick, and sinning. A more applicable Biblical description of those early pioneers would have been Hosea 4:6 — *"My people are destroyed for lack of knowledge."*

Health Conditions in the United States in the 1800's — So lacking was the world in medical knowledge just 150 years ago that the following conditions were commonplace throughout the United States.

- Polluted water supplies.
- Unsanitary means of sewage disposal.
- Unhygienic methods of food preparation and transport.
- No control over mosquitoes, flies, and other insect vectors.
- Rooms were shuttered tight at night because of a fear of night air.
- Sunlight was shunned.
- Women's dresses dragged in the filth of city streets.
- Babies clung to the filth laden hems of their mother's garments or crawled on grimy germ-laden floors.
- Women of high fashion wore the wasp-waist dress, effectively constricting their abdominal organs.
- Men chewed and spit tobacco everywhere.
- The work of Pasteur and Robert Koch that formed the foundation for the germ-theory of disease lay 30 years in the future.

Today, in the United States, infant mortality is less than 1%.[6] In 1875 it was 17%.[7] This means that one out of every six babies failed to reach their first birthday. Nowadays, life expectancy at birth is around 79 years.[8] In 1850 it was 39.4.[9] By 1900 it was still below 50.[10]

The major killers of modern-day society are chronic diseases like heart disease, cancer, stroke, Alzheimer's, and diabetes. One hundred fifty years ago the situation was quite different. Pneumonia, tuberculosis, and dysentery topped the list of assassins. Yellow fever, smallpox, typhoid, diphtheria, measles, cholera, and other third world diseases were equally rampant and devastating.

Malaria — William Rothstein in his historical treatise on nineteenth century medicine makes this almost unbelievable statement, "Malaria was the most common and significant endemic disease in early nineteenth-century America."[11]

Malaria is transmitted by the *Anopheles* mosquito which carries the disease producing protozoa in its saliva. The disease itself is characterized by periods of severe chills and fevers followed by asymptomatic periods. Sometimes there may also be vomiting and severe headaches. It is estimated that worldwide more than 300 million people are afflicted with malaria in any given year.

Parts of the world in which it remains a significant threat include Africa, both Central and South America, and Southeast Asia. A particularly virulent strain is endemic in certain parts of Cambodia, Laos, and northern Thailand.

In December 1998, my family and I went to a small village in northwest Thailand to help build a church during Christmas vacation. Due to a flight delay we missed our connecting flight from Chiang Mai to Mae Hong Son so we spent a day visiting the ancient ruins in Chiang Mai. As we were walking down a street, we passed a government building with a sign in English stating that it was a malaria clinic. Since we had not taken any prophylactics, I went inside hoping to get some information regarding our risk for both malaria and dengue fever. While waiting for assistance, a young man, probably in his twenties, entered. Though outdoor temperatures were in the upper eighties, this man was shaking and shivering uncontrollably, exhibiting telltale signs of malaria.

The disease is virtually unheard of in America today, unless contracted by a traveler returning from the tropics. Yet, 150 years ago it was so prevalent that it was considered a normal part of pioneer life. On at least one occasion, Ellen White herself was afflicted with the disease.[12]

One might have expected it in the marshes of the south, or the undeveloped Western frontier, but it was also a major problem in northern states like Wisconsin and Minnesota. At the time, the cause of malaria was unknown. Not knowing its etiology, most believed that malaria was caused by heavy dews and mists arising out of marshes, swamps, and jungles. The word itself comes from the Latin and means "bad air."

It appears that in her earliest writings on health, Ellen White also held to this popular view of her times. Notice this statement from How to Live which is reprinted in the appendix to Volume II of Selected Messages. *"Dwellings, if possible, should be built upon high and dry ground. If a house be built where water settles around it, remaining for a time, and then drying away, a poisonous miasma arises, and fever and ague* (a word commonly used in her day to describe a malarial attack), *sore throat, lung diseases, and fevers will be the result."*[13]

When similar counsel was given 50 years later in The Ministry of Healing subtle changes in wording took place. *"So far as possible, all buildings intended for human habitation should be placed on high, well-drained ground. This will ensure a dry site and prevent the danger of disease from dampness and miasma. This matter is often too lightly regarded. Continuous ill-health, serious diseases, and many deaths result from the dampness and malaria of low-lying, ill-drained situations."*[14]

At the time of this latter statement mosquitoes were still unknown as the vector in the transmission of malaria. Yet in this latter statement, even though malaria is recognized as occurring more frequently in damp places, the environmental "miasma" as a causal factor is toned down compared to the earlier statement. I believe this illustrates how Ellen White herself, not having a medical background, had to grow in her understanding of health and disease.

Other endemic diseases of America during the 1800's included diarrheal diseases, especially dysentery, commonly called the "*flux or bloody flux.*" This disease is characterized by fever, cramps, and a bloody, mucous diarrhea. Due to current sanitation efforts directed towards food and water supplies, it too is virtually unknown today in the United States. However, in third-world developing countries it continues to be a challenge and is a primary cause of infant mortality.

Respiratory diseases, namely pneumonia, influenza, and tuberculosis, were also major causes of illness and death. In 1894, one public health official estimated that as many as one quarter of the adult population in the United States died from tuberculosis alone.[15] On a percentage basis, that is equivalent to the number dying from cancer today.

Numerous epidemics added to the burden of the above diseases. Plagues of cholera, yellow fever, diphtheria, typhoid, and smallpox struck communities with such abruptness and high mortality that "the effects could only be compared to the effects of warfare in the twentieth century."[16]

Cholera — Of the numerous contagious diseases, cholera seems to have been the most devastating. Major epidemics occurred in 1832, 1849–1854, and 1866. In the 1854 epidemic in New York City, on at least two occasions the morning shift physicians discovered that during the night not only had all the patients on the cholera ward died, but so had all the nurses treating them.[17] Thus was the rapidity with which cholera could strike.

This is another example of a disease from which the Whites were not spared. At the time James began to publish the *Advent Review* he suffered a severe bout of cholera; so severe that Ellen was afraid he might die.[18]

The 1852 epidemic struck Rochester, New York while the Whites were living there. Mrs. White wrote in her diary that through the night she could hear carriages rumbling along the streets as they bore the dead to Mount Hope Cemetery. At this time, their three-year-old son was afflicted. It was only in answer to prayer that Edson made a miraculous recovery.

Yellow Fever and Diphtheria — Between 1800 and 1879, major outbreaks of yellow fever appeared every year except two. In the devastating epidemic of 1793 that hit Philadelphia, 4,000 out of 27,000 residents died.[19] The magnitude of the destruction caused by this outbreak was particularly frightening since Philadelphia was the capital of the United States at the time and many government officials actually fled the city.

Diphtheria was the bane of children. It is characterized by a severe sore throat and the formation of a membrane across the larynx that causes suffocation. Often several children in the same family would die during an epidemic.

Serious illness was thus a major part of the lives of Americans. Even the most rudimentary understanding of infection was lacking as physicians knew nothing of the role of bacteria or viruses as causal agents. They were unable to diagnose most diseases and could only try to treat symptoms.

The belief in disease being either a punishment of God or an affliction from Satan had carried over from the Dark Ages. Not knowing any other cause for her husband's sickness, Ellen blamed James' bout with cholera on Satan's efforts to hinder the work. The same reasoning was exhibited when Edson contracted the same disease. "We believed the affliction of the child was the work of Satan, to hinder us from traveling" (in evangelistic efforts).[20]

Bleeding As a Cure — In such a milieu of medical ignorance, two major schools of medical treatment emerged, bleeding and drugging. Bleeding or bloodletting was based on the symptomatic treatment of the day. During sickness it was observed that frequently the patient was feverish, with rapid heart rate, and flushed face. This was assumed to be the result of too much blood. So the obvious cure was to decrease the amount of blood. In this treatment one can see the carryover effects of Greek thought that taught the need to balance the humours in the body.

The dominant thinking advocated bleeding until syncope or unconsciousness. This was seen as indicative that the right quantity of blood had been removed. Sometimes this meant withdrawing copious amounts. Medical reports of the day are replete with case studies. As you read the following two accounts cited by Rothstein, keep in mind that on average the adult human body contains about five liters or one and a quarter gallons of blood.

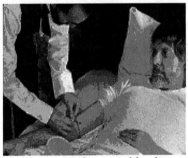

19th century physician bleeding a patient

"Before he arrived Dr. Colby had made preparations for bleeding her, thinking prompt blood-letting necessary, and that a high peritoneal inflammation existed. Dr. Drake concurred, and they proceeded to bleed. When six or eight ounces were abstracted, Dr. Colby, thinking she had been bled as much as her constitution would bear, ...arrested the flow of blood. Dr. Drake was much dissatisfied, and insisted on a more copious bleeding. The bandage was accordingly removed, and more blood taken. It was then replaced. Dr. Drake still remained unsatisfied, urging that it was necessary to bleed to fainting. The difference of opinion was presented to the family, and Dr. Richards was brought in. Drs. Richards and Drake both soon agreed as to the necessity of bleeding, and she

was again bled... Forty grains of calomel were then admin-
istered. Thirty ounces of blood had been taken. Still Drs.
Drake and Richards were not satisfied -- they thought fur-
ther bleeding was necessary, yet postponed it till morning.

[The next morning.] All the symptoms boded well. But
Drs. Drake and Richards were of the opinion that she had
not been bled sufficiently. They accordingly recommended
further bleeding; Dr. Colby opposed it,... [A fourth phy-
sician, Dr. Eberle, was sent for.] He concurred with the
majority, and further bleeding was consequently resolved
upon. It was anticipated that the effect would be to reduce
the frequency of the pulse, and augment its volume! Kitty
was told that the doctor thought of bleeding her again, and
was asked if she was willing. She said "Yes, anything." She
was then raised up in bed, and twenty ounces of blood were
taken from her. The effect on the pulse was the exact con-
trary of what was anticipated. It became more frequent and
more feeble, but in other respects she seemed somewhat
easier. The physicians seemed to entertain some hopes of
her recovery, and agreed upon a course of treatment to be
adopted. The [patient's] father came into [her] room ex-
claiming, "Thank God, my child, the doctors say there is
hope." She said nothing. All hope had vanished....Dr. Drake
felt her pulse, and said she was dead."

The second case which involved the same Dr. Colby
has a more amusing ending.

"Old Dr. Colby was in the habit of getting his lancet out
and laying it upon the table before even removing his hat,
or before ascertaining what the disease might be that he
was called to see. Bleeding was done in any event. It was
all part of the routine of practice.... Bleeding was primary,
first and foremost in all cases and condition. I remember
that a horse kicked me once as Dr. Colby was passing the
house. I was not injured much, yet mother called in the
doctor, and he at once proceeded to bleed me-- I presume on
general principles. I had seen my mother bled a great many
times. The doctor would always bleed her sitting up in the
bed, and when she would faint and fall over in the bed he
loosened the bandages. The doctor had me sitting upon the

bed, and when a small quantity of blood escaped, I shut my eyes and fell over on the bed. I remember he told mother that he never saw any one so speedily affected by bleeding. This was the only time I ever was bled."[21]

Death of George Washington — Even George Washington, the first president of the United States, was bled to death. We know this because his doctors kept accurate notes on their treatment so that the American populace would be assured that their former president had received the best medical care available.

On a cold, wet wintry day in December, Washington spent several hours working outside on his farm at Mount Vernon. That night he came down with a fever and severe sore throat. The following evening, as his condition began to worsen, he instructed one of his overseers to bleed him. Later, when his personal physician arrived, he was bled some more. Later still, upon the arrival of a consulting physician, more blood was extracted. By the time Washington pled with his doctors to "let me go quietly," some 80 ounces of blood had been removed in 12 hours.[22] This was equal to about 35% of the total blood in his body. In addition he was blistered, and vomited, and purged with tartar emetic and calomel.

Even the six foot two inch robust former President could not endure this treatment. Fortunately for Americans who revere George Washington as "The Father of Their Country," he had been able to endure those diseases which frequently struck down weaker individuals. Historical records show that from age seventeen he experienced several recurrences of malaria, diphtheria, smallpox which left him scarred for life, tuberculosis and pleurisy, three bouts of dysentery, and severely infected tonsils.[23] Many historians conclude that it was his doctors' intervention during his last illness that hastened his demise on December 14, 1799 at the age of 67.

Use of Poisonous Drugs — The other dominant medical practice was drugging. Two categories of drugs were used: emetics which induced vomiting, and cathartics or purgatives, that worked as powerful laxatives.

In the 18th century, calomel, a chloride of mercury, was introduced as a drug to clean out the bowels. As a therapeutic agent it is useless. However, in the intestine it breaks down into highly poisonous components, which then irritate and purge. For physicians who believed in drugging, calomel was almost as important as bleeding.

It gained notoriety in the United States during the 1793 yellow fever epidemic in Philadelphia, when its most noted physician, Dr. Benjamin Rush, used it extensively and massively in treating victims. So debilitating were its effects that it is likely that more yellow fever victims died at the hands of Dr. Rush than from the disease itself.[24]

"Tartar Emetic" produced vomiting. In large doses, it lowered the pulse and body temperature. It was also a lethal poison. Another popular purgative was Nitre, or salt-peter, which like tartar emetic depressed the heart-beat. And like tartar emetic, it was deadly poisonous.

One can only imagine the debilitating and dehydrating effects such potent drugs had on a patient. Once the body had been cleansed of excessive fluids and the fever was reduced, tonics were administered with the purpose of building up the system through improved appetite and good digestion. One of the most popular tonics was arsenic. After the Civil War it was replaced by quinine and later strychnine. The most important tonic though and probably the most important medicinal agent was beverage alcohol, almost always in the form of whiskey or brandy. Alcohol was used in both acute and chronic diseases, foremost among the former being typhoid and pneumonia.

After bacteriology became a science, it was discovered that alcohol acted as a germicide, effectively killing bacteria on contact. From this it was deducted that alcohol would also kill bacteria if taken internally. So by the end of the century the use of beverage alcohol as a medicinal actually increased.

Then there were the analgesics of which opium and its alkaloid, morphine, were the most important. Opium was used by physicians in every conceivable illness. It was probably the most common treatment for diarrhea but physicians also prescribed it for fevers, inflammations, and aches and pains of all kinds. In 1888, a survey indicated that opium was in 14 percent of all prescriptions written.[25] Enormous amounts of opium were imported into the United States, spawning a rapidly growing addiction to the drug. Before the Civil War, Dr. Worthington Hooker wrote that " Opium...is the most important of all drugs that are employed in the treatment of disease."[26]

Considering the times, one can readily understand why Ellen White wrote so vehemently against drug therapy. *"I was shown that the innocent, modest-looking, white poppy yields a dangerous drug. Opium is a slow poison, when taken in small quantities. In large doses it produces lethargy and death. Its effects upon the nervous system are ruinous. When patients use this drug until it becomes habit, it is almost impossible to discontinue it...*

The opium slave is in a pitiful condition. Unless his nervous system is continually intoxicated with the poisonous drug, he is miserable. It benumbs the sensibilities, stupefies the brain, and unfits the mind for the service of God. True Christians cannot persist in the use of this slow poison, when they know its influence upon them.

...God is displeased that his followers should become slaves to habits which ruin body and mind. Nux vomica, or strychnine, and opium have killed their millions, and have left thousands upon the earth to linger out a wretched, suffering existence, a burden to themselves, and those around them.

Mercury, calomel, and quinine have brought their amount of wretchedness, which the day of God alone will fully reveal. Preparations of mercury and calomel taken into the system ever retain their poisonous strength as long as there is a particle of it left in the system. These poisonous preparations have destroyed their millions, and left sufferers upon the earth to linger out a miserable existence. All are better off without these dangerous mixtures. Miserable sufferers, with disease in almost every form, misshapen by suffering, with dreadful ulcers, and pains in the bones, loss of teeth, loss of memory, and impaired sight, are to be seen almost every where. They are victims of poisonous preparations, which have been, in many cases, administered to cure some slight indisposition, which after a day or two of fasting would have disappeared without medicine. But poisonous mixtures, administered by physicians, have proved their ruin.

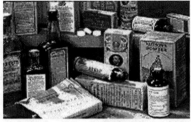

...God's servants should not administer medicines which they know will leave behind injurious effects upon the system, even if they do relieve present suffering."[27]

Distribution of medicines was hardly regulated at all. After the Civil War, quackery became big business and flourished until the early 20th century. Richard Schaeffer in <u>Legacy</u> gives a list of some of these pseudo-medicines, including *Kickapoo Indian Remedies, Ponzzoni's Complexion Powder, Mrs. Winslow's Soothing Syrup, White Star Secret Liquor Cure, La Dore's Bust Food, Dr. Killmer's Swamp Root, Dr. Pierce's Pleasant Pellets,* and my favorite sounding one, *Dr. William's Pink Pills for Pale People.*[28]

No wonder a cartoonist of the day depicted a physician wondering, "Why the devil does it happen that all my patients succumb? I bleed them well, drug them, purge them. I simply cannot understand."

Men like Oliver Wendall Holmes recognized the futility of it all. *"If the whole materia medica, as now used, could be sunk to the bottom of the sea, it would be all the better for mankind — and all the worse for the fishes."*[29]

It is really difficult to imagine the terrible effects these commonly administered treatments had on their patients. One would have had to live in those days to realize the terrible character of regular medicine. Patients were unwashed. Clothing and bedding went days without being changed. Dirty and malodorous, the afflicted were tormented continuously with nausea and terrible thirst inflicted by bleeding, blisters, purging, and cathartics that were prescribed in almost every case of illness.

The mortality was large, ranging from ten to fifty per cent. Many refused to call the physician if it were possible to avoid doing so and thereby often increased their chances of recovery. Nor was it just the poor, uneducated, ignorant classes who suffered. Reference has already been made to the death of President Washington. And the above mentioned Kitty, who died at the age of twenty-three while being treated for puerperal fever, undoubtedly caused by the dirty hands of the physicians who delivered her baby, was the first wife of Salmon Chase, who later became governor of Ohio and was secretary of the treasury during the Lincoln presidency. Delving into the medical texts available, Salmon became convinced that his wife would not have died had she not been bled so profusely. He soon remarried but his second, and then his third wife also died in the prime of life. And the child that Kitty had given birth to? She lived only five years before succumbing to an epidemic of scarlet fever. When some years later his favorite sister, Hannah, had a fatal heart attack during dinner, Governor Chase lamented, "Death has pursued me incessantly since I was twenty-five."[30]

Shortly after graduating from medical school in 1835, J. Marion Sims, who later became a noted gynecologist, wrote, *"The practice of that time was heroic: it was murderous. I knew nothing about medicine, but I had sense enough to see that doctors were killing their patients, that medicine was not an exact science, that it was wholly empirical and that it would be better to trust entirely to Nature than to the hazardous skill of the doctors."*[31]

What I have portrayed here is but a dim picture of medicine in the United States of America just 150 years ago. Normal occupations consisted of caring for the sick and burying the dead. Torrential tears of anguish and pain flowed from souls desperate for healing while knowing that they were dying without the hope of ever finding it.

Many believed their afflictions were due to some evil in their lives and thousands begged mercy from heaven.

As has been noted, the pioneers of Adventism also endured the agony and anguish of those days. They too suffered an unfair amount of blood, drugs, and tears. But, they believed they had an important calling; a divine mission. That mission was to proclaim the Three Angels' messages; messages designed to prepare a remnant people for the imminent return of Jesus Christ.

But how could they proclaim that message when they were bedridden much of the time? How could they carry that message to the far corners of the earth, when they themselves were dying in the prime of youth and early adulthood?

We serve a loving God; a God who wants His people to be free from pain, and sorrow, and suffering. In his mercy, God looked down upon the United States of America and a small band of committed Christians who were forming the nucleus of His remnant people. And out of that relatively small circle of believers, he took the sickest of the sick, and the weakest of the weak, and gave to her a message that was literally a life saver to His saints.

But it was more than that. For when rightly understood, the message of health, hope, and healing that God has given to Seventh-day Adventists is a message of restoration and redemption. It is a message that needs to be lived out in the lives of Seventh-day Adventists today. And it is a message that needs to be proclaimed boldly to the world. When followed in its completeness, it is a message that restores mankind into the image of God — physically, mentally, and above all, spiritually. It is imperative then that we understand the components of that message.

CHAPTER 5

VISION OF HEALTH, HOPE, AND HEALING

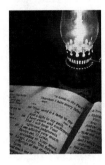

And it shall come to pass in the last days, that I will pour out my Spirit on all flesh; and your sons and your daughters shall prophesy, Your young men shall see visions, Your old men shall dream dreams.

And on My menservants and on My maidservants I will pour out My Spirit in those days; and they shall prophesy.

Acts 2:17, 18

July 1863 — Gettysburg, Pennsylvania — The United States was in the midst of a terrible Civil War. It was a conflict in which more American fathers, sons, and husbands would be killed than in any other war. Various figures indicate between 560,000 and 618,000 American soldiers died during its four years from 1861–1865. However, two thirds of the fatalities were caused by disease and contagion rather than from gunshot wounds

The army camps were overcrowded, squalid quagmires of dirt and vermin. Often the tents were pitched near mosquito infested muddy swamps. Food was of a poor quality; even rotten at times. Antibiotics were nonexistent. Sanitation and sterile procedures were unknown. T. Longmore, the 1863 author of <u>A Treatise on Gunshot</u>

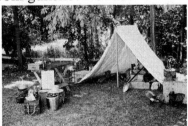

A Civil War campsite

Wounds wrote, "Of all instruments for conducting an examination of a gunshot wound, the finger of the surgeon is most appropriate."[1]

In almost 100% of the cases, that finger would have been ungloved; unwashed; unclean. While working on the field of battle, surgeons never bothered to stop to wash from their hands the blood of a wounded man; nor to clean off their clothes before moving on to the next patient. Even their surgical instruments were washed only once — at the end of the day. Sometimes the same bandages were used on multiple patients without any sort of cleansing in between.

No wonder epidemics of diarrhea, dysentery, measles, mumps, pneumonia, and typhoid fever were as much of a dirge as enemy bullets. One doctor spoke proudly of the fact that it was only two out of three who died from disease. Bad as this number sounds, it represented a 25% drop from the Mexican-American War just 15 years earlier when seven out of eight had died from illness.[2]

In terms of actual battlefield casualties, the costliest battle was fought at Gettysburg during the first three days of July 1863 in which as many as 51,000 were killed, wounded, or missing in action; the climax occurring with the massive slaughter on the final day of the battle.

Gettysburg was a small town situated in the midst of farmlands covering the southeastern Pennsylvania landscape. Militarily it was insignificant. As a matter of fact, the confrontation that started just north of the city happened unexpectedly.

The rebellious confederate Army of Northern Virginia under the command of General Robert E. Lee, had up to this point won almost every major battle with the North. General Lee believed it was time to make an all out assault on the capital, Washington D.C. His strategy called for a sweeping run through the Pennsylvania farmlands before attacking from the less protected northern side of the city. The plan would also enable him to replenish his dwindling food supplies.

On July 1, advance troops were reconnoitering along the Chambersburg Pike west of the city. In the approaching light of dawn they fired at a Union cavalry soldier who was spying upon them. The battle that became the turning point of the American Civil War had begun.

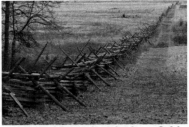

Split rail fence lined wheat field where thousands were slain in the battle of Gettysburg

For two and a half days fierce fighting continued. The tide swayed back and forth; first favoring the South, then the North, and back again to the South. In their trenches south of town, Union forces courageously repelled assault after assault of rebel attacks against their flanks.

In the early afternoon of the third day of battle, General Lee felt that his opponents had been sufficiently weakened to launch a final assault aimed at victory. The two armies faced each other along two high ridges. West of Emmitsburg Road, Lee's men held the high ground of Seminary Ridge. General Meade's troops were dug in along Cemetery Ridge. Between the two armies lay a wide open expanse known as the "wheat field."

Beginning at precisely 1:00 pm and continuing for two hours, a deafening artillery barrage rang out from both sides of the valley. The cannonade was so intense that the editors of a <u>Civil War Times Illustrated</u> document entitled *Gettysburg*, called it "the most stupendous artillery duel ever witnessed on the American continent."[3] When the firing ceased, General George Pickett was ordered to begin his now infamous charge.

Thirteen thousand strong came the attack. Down Seminary Ridge, across the open fields; in column after column, with battle flags fluttering in the breeze the infantrymen marched toward impending doom. As they neared the Emmitsburg Road, they had to pause to batter down the sturdy farm fences lining the road. Without warning a hellish bombardment rained down upon them with deadly accuracy from the Union cannons and muskets.

Within moments the road and surrounding fields turned crimson as one man after another was mowed down, caught in the murderous onslaught. Helplessly the Confederate batteries atop Seminary Ridge watched the devastation befalling their brave comrades. Their cannons sat idle for fear that firing them would wreak additional havoc on their own troops as they neared hand-to-hand combat with the enemy.

Sheer willpower enabled some of the rebel troops to penetrate the Union line, but they were quickly rebuffed. Those who remained limped back to the safety of Seminary Ridge. In the no-man's land of the wheat field, thousands of Confederate soldiers lay dead and wounded. The back of the Southern forces had been broken. And though General Lee would continue to fight on for almost two more years, he never again experienced the string of victories that had been his leading up to Gettysburg.

The American Civil War finally ended on April 9, 1865 when General Robert E. Lee handed over his battle sword to Union General Ulysses S. Grant and signed a declaration of surrender at Appomattox Courthouse in the state of Virginia. One week later, President Abraham Lincoln, sought an evening of relaxation from the pressures that had been his during the four years of war. While watching a play at Ford's Theater, he was shot in the back of the head by an assassin, John Wilkes Booth. America now faced a dark and uncertain future.

Adventism's Beginnings — At the time the Battle of Gettysburg took place, the fledgling Seventh-day Advent movement had been in existence for less than 20 years. On October 22, 1844, more than 50,000 in the Northeastern United States alone believed that before the day was finished, Jesus would return to earth in His glorious second coming. But on October 23, the morning after the Great Disappointment, that number had dwindled to no more than a few handfuls. The others had either given up on the Bible and Christianity, or they returned to the nominal churches of the day, embarrassed that they had got caught up in the "fanaticism" of the Millerite movement.

The small nucleus that remained was comprised of ardent students of the Bible. They believed that according to Biblical prophecy, something significant had indeed happened on October 22. So they studied and prayed and studied some more. Their meeting places were houses, barns, stables, and even cornfields. Under the leadership of James and Ellen White, and Joseph Bates, that small nucleus grew, until in 1863 there were 3,500 Advent believers; enough to make up several conferences. For further growth to occur it was important that there be some sort of formal organization. Thus on May 21, 1863, just 6 weeks prior to the Battle of Gettysburg, the General Conference of Seventh-day Adventists was formerly organized with its headquarters in Battle Creek, Michigan.

On a Friday evening, just two weeks after the Church's formal organization, the Whites found themselves in the home of brother Hilliard in Otsego, Michigan. Along with several other wagons they had traveled the 25 miles northwestward from Battle Creek in order to lend their

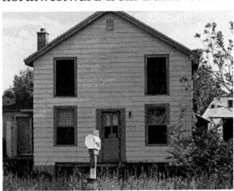

support to evangelistic meetings being held by R. J. Lawrence and M. E. Cornell.[4]

There was a secondary reason for the Whites' trip to Otsego. Though only 41-years-old, James was suffering telltale signs of burnout from "constant and excessive labor." It was hoped that he could get away for a few days for some much needed rest.

The Hilliard house where Ellen White received her comprehensive health vision is still standing today.

As the Hilliard's and their visitors engaged in sundown worship that Friday evening, Mrs.White was asked to lead in prayer. Her deep burden was that James' health would be restored. While praying she moved across the room to his side and placed her hand on his shoulder. It was then that she was taken off in vision which lasted about 45 minutes. This vision is now known as the "Comprehensive Health Reform Vision" because of the instruction given during that time. To this day it forms the basis for the primary tenets of the Adventist Church's teachings on health. The complete account as written in the summer of 1864 covered 10 categories of counsel and can be found in <u>Spiritual Gifts, Vol. 4.</u>

Components of the Comprehensive Health Vision —

1. **Care of Health as a Religious Duty** — *"I saw that it was a sacred duty to attend to our health, and arouse others to their duty.... All are required to do what they can to preserve healthy bodies and sound minds."*[5]

2. **The Cause of Disease Is a Violation of Health Laws** — *"Many are living in violation of the laws of health, and are ignorant of the relation their habits of eating, drinking, and working sustain to their health."*[6]

3. **Intemperance in Every Form Is to be Shunned** — *"Tobacco in whatever form it is used is a slow poison."*[7] *"It is a poison of the most deceitful and malignant kind."*[8] *"God is displeased that his followers should become slaves to habits which ruin body and mind. Nux vomica, or strychnine, and opium have killed their millions.... Mercury, calomel, and quinine have brought their amount of wretchedness, which the day of God alone will fully reveal."*[9]

4. **Vegetarianism Is the Ideal Diet** — *"God gave our first parents the food He designed that the race should eat. It was contrary to His plan to have the life of any creature be taken."*[10]

5. **Regularity in Eating Habits** — *"Indulging in eating too frequently, and in too large quantities, over-taxes the digestive organs, and produces a feverish state of the system. The blood becomes impure, and then diseases of various kinds occur."*[11]

6. **The Role of the Mind in Sickness and Health** — *"There is a class of invalids who have no real located disease. But as they believe they are dangerously diseased, they are in reality invalids. The mind is diseased, and many die who might recover of disease, which exists alone in the imagination."*[12]

7. **Natural Remedies in Healing** — *"Drugs never cure disease....Nature alone has curative powers."*[13]

8. **Personal Cleanliness** — *"I have been shown that a great amount of suffering might be saved if all would labor to prevent disease, by strictly obeying the laws of health. Strict habits of cleanliness should be observed."*[14]

9. **Environmental Concerns** — *"Every family that prizes health should cleanse their houses and their premises of all decaying substances."*[15]

10. **Health Education by the Church** — *"I saw that it was a sacred duty to attend to our health and to arouse others to their duty."*[16]

There they are—ten laws of life designed to preserve and protect the human mechanism. It is interesting to note, that just as God gave ten commandments to ancient Israel in the desert, so He gave ten principles for healthy living to the Adventist church in its early wilderness experience. It is also interesting to compare these principles with the basic tenets of the Mosaic Health Code as presented in Chapter 2.

Think of how radical these teachings must have sounded 150 years ago. Remember, the majority believed that diseases were caused by some miasma that permeated the night air. The "heroic" medical practices of bleeding and drugging, primary treatments prescribed for almost every disease, were more likely to kill patients than cure them. Even tobacco was recommended for lung diseases.

Concepts of cleanliness and sanitation were virtually non-existent. Daily bathing was unheard of. Elder James Nix, curator of the Ellen White Estate, tells of how James White, after one of his many trips was glad to return home and be able to take the first bath that he had had in several weeks.[17] Spitting along city streets was common. The skirts of women of fashion dragged in the dusty filth of those same streets.

The sciences of nutrition and biochemistry were in their infancy. Vitamins had yet to be discovered. Meat, potatoes, lard, and hard biscuits were the daily fare. Science had not yet vindicated the importance of a diet rich in fruits, vegetables, and unrefined grains.

So when Ellen White penned the above 10-tenet program for good health, much of it appeared to be radical when compared with the mainstream medical positions of her time. The world renown Dr. John Harvey Kellogg wrote the preface to a compilation of some of Ellen White's earliest writings on health. In it he stated the following: *"At the time the writings first appeared, the subject of health was almost wholly ignored, not only by the people to whom they were addressed, but by the world at large."*[18]

He went on to say, *"Nowhere and by no one was there presented a systematic and harmonious body of hygienic truths, free from patent errors and consistent with the Bible.... The principles taught were not enforced by scientific authority, but were presented in a simple, straightforward manner by one who makes no pretense to scientific knowledge, but claims to write by the aid and authority of the divine enlightenment."*[19]

Thus early Adventists had to accept the health message on the basis of faith. With our increased scientific knowledge and understanding, may I suggest that Seventh-day Adventists today have no excuse for following through on this knowledge. Yet how often we fail. How often I fail.

Health Reform Movements of the 1800's — Without a doubt, the words penned in <u>Spiritual Gifts, Vol. IV</u> one hundred and forty years ago, are just as timely now as they were then. However, in order to maintain historical honesty, one needs to understand that Ellen White was not the originator of these concepts or principles. Since the 1830's the medical schools of Europe had been abandoning bleeding and drugging as ineffectual remedies. Simultaneously various health reform movements were springing up in America.

For example there was a proliferation of vegetarian societies. One of America's founding fathers and a signer of The Declaration of Independence, Benjamin Franklin, tells in his <u>Autobiography</u> of how he contemplated starting a church based on adherence to a vegetarian diet and keeping the seventh-day Sabbath.[20]

An even stronger advocate of vegetarianism was Sylvester Graham. A Presbyterian minister, he toured widely, emphasizing a natural foods diet utilizing stone ground unbolted wheat or rye flour. In his memory, Graham Crackers are named after him.

Graham also railed against alcohol, tobacco, tea, coffee, spices, excess sexual activity and masturbation. He promoted the use of water, both internally and externally, encouraged physical activity, and denounced the tight fitting corsets worn by women of the period. However, after his death in 1851, the health practices that he had emphasized began to die out, with perhaps the exception of the water cures or hydropathy as they were known.

Drs. Joel Shew and Russell Trall were the primary pioneers in hydropathy. (Kellogg, who studied under Trall, is credited with having renamed water treatments as "hydrotherapy.") The hydrotherapy movement actually began in Austria with a farm boy, Vincent Priessnitz. Due to the success of his treatments, water-cure spas sprung up all over Europe.

In 1843, Joel Shew opened America's first water-cure center in New York City. Two years later he began publishing the *Water-Cure Journal*. Over the next half century more than 200 hydropathy centers opened and eventually the *Water-Cure Journal* reached a circulation of almost one hundred thousand.[21]

Perhaps hydropathy would have never reached its level of prominence though, had it not been for Russell Trall, M.D. Although trained in allopathic methods he had little regard for the regular medical practices of the day. In an attempt to find cures that had less cruel side effects, he experimented with both herbal and homeopathic alternatives. But it was hydropathy, which he preferred to call "hygiotherapy," that really caught his attention. When in 1867 he opened "The Hygeian Home" along the Delaware River in rural New Jersey, it instantly became one of the nation's most sought after havens of health.

Another practicing physician who gained notoriety through his water-cure facility was James Caleb Jackson, M.D. It was to his "Our Home on the Hillside" in Dansville, New York that Ellen White brought her husband for recovery from his stroke in 1865.[22]

In 1848, Larkin B. Coles, a physician from Boston, published Philosophy of Health, a manual that presented simple rules for healthful living in easily understood language. In some of her early writings, Ellen White borrowed extensively from his writings as they best seemed to express the concepts the Lord had shown her in vision.

In fact, readers who are aware of many of the health teachings promoted in such works as How to Live and The Ministry of Healing may be astounded by the similarity between the teachings in these books and those advocated by men like Larkin, Trall, and Graham. Ellen White herself admits to the similarities in her teachings. She also confesses to having some of the writings of these other authorities in her home. To avoid charges of plagiarism she describes how she first wrote out the health reform vision before consulting these other writings.

The editor of the *Advent Review and Sabbath Herald* asks a question regarding the Comprehensive Vision. — "Did you receive your views upon health reform before visiting the Health Institute at Dansville, New York, or before you had read works on the subject?"

Answer — *"I did not visit Dansville till August, 1864, fourteen months after I had the view. I did not read any works upon health until I had written Spiritual Gifts, Volumes 3 and 4, Appeal to Mothers, and had sketched out most of my six articles in the six numbers of How to Live.*

I did not know that such a paper existed as The Laws of Life, published at Dansville, N.Y. I had not heard of the several works upon health, written by Dr. J. C. Jackson, and other publications at Dansville, at the time I had the view named above. I did not know that such works existed until September, 1863, when in Boston, Mass., my husband saw them advertised in a periodical called The Voice of the Prophets, published by Eld. J. V. Himes. My husband ordered the works from Dansville and received them at Topsham, Maine. His business gave him no time to peruse them, and as I determined not to read them until I had written out my views, the books remained in their wrappers.

As I introduced the subject of health to friends where I labored in Michigan, New England, and in the State of New York, and spoke against drugs and flesh meats, and in favor of water, pure air, and a proper diet, the reply was often made, "You speak very nearly the opinions taught in the Laws of Life, and other publications, by Drs. Trall, Jackson, and others. Have you read that paper and those works?"

My reply was that I had not, neither should I read them till I had fully written out my views, lest it should be said that I have received my light upon the subject of health from physicians, and not from the Lord.

And after I had written my six articles for How to Live, I then searched the various works on hygiene and was surprised to find them so nearly in harmony with what the

Lord had revealed to me. And to show this harmony, and to set before my brethren and sisters the subject as brought out by able writers, I determined to publish How to Live, in which I largely extracted from the works referred to."[23]

In 1868, Dr. Trall was invited to give a week of lectures to the Adventist ministers at Battle Creek. During this time he was a guest of the Whites. As they rode together to the meeting place, Ellen White would share her views on hygiene, disease and its causes, and medicine. At the end of the second day, Dr. Trall asked Mrs. White from what medical school she had graduated, so in harmony were her statements with sound medical science. By the end of the week he wanted to know why He had been invited to speak since, "Mrs. White is just as well prepared to give them the needed instruction on hygiene, as I am."[24]

It should not escape notice either that as the problems of the American Civil War overtook the United States, many of the early reform movements were lost sight of. Historians note that survival issues associated with the Civil War effectually brought to an end the alternative options promoted through the popular health reform movement of the 1830's through the 1850's.

Many institutions that managed to struggle through the war years closed shortly after. For example, two of the White boys, along with Merritt and John Harvey Kellogg, studied at Trall's Hygio-Therapeutic College. But after they completed the course it closed down. In addition, the American Medical Society was founded in 1847 with the intent of suppressing competition from any forms of treatment other than its own allopathic methods.

Thus it was at a very critical moment in history that God spoke in vision to Ellen White on June 6, 1863. But there is something else about the timing of the vision that I think is noteworthy.

Parallels Between Ancient Israel and Early Adventism — Like the early Adventist pioneers, the ancient Israelites were not a healthy lot when they left Egypt. Sickness and ill-health had been rampant in the country of their bondage. So upon their deliverance, the first message that God gave them was a health message.

Look up Exodus 15. The first twenty verses contain the Song of Miriam, a song of deliverance and praise. Then there is the experience of the bitter waters at Marah. Just before the chapter concludes, verse 26 records the first words of instruction from the Lord after the crossing of the Red Sea. It is this verse upon which chapter two of this book is predicated.

"If you diligently heed the voice of the Lord your God, and do what is right in His sight, give ear to His commandments, and keep all His statutes, I will put none of the diseases upon you which I have brought on the Egyptians. For I am the Lord who heals you."

Now come back to the 1800's. On May 21, 1863, the Seventh-day Adventist Church was officially organized. Again, the first instruction that God gave for the edification and redemption of His people after that significant event was the "Comprehensive Health Message." Evidently as far as God is concerned, there is a close correlation between obedience to the physical laws of health and spiritual progress towards the Promised Land.

Paul understood this correlation. Notice how clear he makes it in Romans 12:1, 2 — *"I beseech you therefore, brethren, by the mercies of God, that you present your bodies, a living sacrifice, holy, acceptable to God, which is your reasonable service. And do not be confirmed to this world but be transformed by the renewing of your mind, that you may prove what is that good and acceptable and perfect will of God."*

In the ancient Jewish sacrificial system, the repentant sinner had to offer a lamb without spot or blemish for atonement for sin. This lamb of course represented the death of the spotless Son of God as an atonement for our sins. Paul draws from this symbolism to plead with the Christians in Rome to live lives fully committed to God. He challenges them to depart from the practices of the world around them. Notice the phraseology.

"Present your bodies a living sacrifice."
"Be not confirmed to this world."
"Renew your mind."

Here is presented the Scriptural basis for the Adventist emphasis on a threefold education — body, mind, and spirit. Here is the basis for the Seventh-day Adventist health work. Elder J. H. Waggoner understood this intimate connection when he wrote in the *Review and Herald* of August 7, 1866:

"...when placed on a level with the great truths of the third angel's messages by the sanction and authority of God's spirit, and so declared to be the means whereby a weak people may be made strong to overcome, and our diseased bodies cleansed and fitted for translation, then it comes to us as an essential part of present truth, to be received with the blessing of God, or rejected at our peril."

Formal church organization and an enlightened emphasis on healthful living occurred almost simultaneously. The impact of that comprehensive health vision and subsequent visions on similar topics, was so great that just three years later, in the fall of 1866, the fledgling Seventh-day Adventist Church opened the doors to its first health care facility, the Western Health Reform Institute. This became the forerunner to the world famous Battle Creek Sanitarium. The growth of that institution literally propelled Seventh-day Adventists into the national limelight.

CHAPTER 6

GOD SENT A MAN

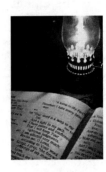

...who knows whether you have come to the kingdom for such a time as this?

Esther 4:14

March 20, 1997 — Los Angeles, California — The tone was gruff and adamant, "Lady, what are you doing in here?"

Startled, my wife turned around and came face-to-face with a tall imposing individual. On his sleeve he wore the insignia of a United States of America immigration officer.

We had been in Hong Kong for several years when Loma Linda University announced it was hosting the 2nd International Congress on Vegetarianism. Since Mieko had a Master's degree in Nutrition, we decided this would be a good opportunity for her to catch up on the latest findings in her field.

However, upon arrival at Los Angeles International airport, she was faced with an unexpected problem. Just weeks before embarking on this trip, she had renewed her Japanese passport. All of her official records regarding previous travel to and from the United States, as well as her reentry permit were in her old passport. And that passport had been left behind in a dresser drawer in our apartment. Without it, United States immigration had the authority to send her back to Hong Kong on the next flight.

What to do? A quick prayer to heaven's courts for divine intervention and Mieko found herself being directed to the airport immigration office. Fortunately this was in the days before 9/11 or the outcome might have been different.

Finding a room with a placard reading "United States Immigration Service," she lightly knocked on the half ajar door.

No response.

She pushed the door open a bit further as she called out, "Hello? Excuse me! Excuse me! Is anyone here?"

Still no answer.

So she entered and looked around while continuing to call, "Hello? Is anyone here?"

It was then that she heard the intimidating voice behind her, "Lady, what are you doing here! You are not allowed to enter this room!"

With trepidation, Mieko turned around to see an immense figure blocking the door. Trembling she poured out her story; how she had left her old passport with documentation back in Hong Kong; how she had come all this way to attend a conference; how the immigration officer at the customs desk had directed her to this office; and how she now needed his help to continue with her trip.

"What are you doing in Hong Kong?" was his first question.

Mieko replied. "I'm working in a hospital as an overseas worker for my church."

"Which hospital?" The tone was still skeptical.

Mieko began to wonder where this line of questioning was leading. "Why does he want to know which hospital? Rather than solving my problem, why is he asking for the name of the hospital where I am working? Besides he has probably never heard of Seventh-day Adventists and so will ask me a lot more questions." But rather than expressing these thoughts, she answered, "Hong Kong Adventist Hospital."

"Are you Adventist?" The tone of voice was becoming softer, more congenial.

"Yes, I am a Seventh-day Adventist," Mieko quickly answered.

"Well lady, so am I." Then he said something that left Mieko stunned. "I was transferred to this post less than two weeks ago. I think the Lord sent me here to help you." And then he stamped the proper entry permit into her passport, thereby authorizing her stay.

Throughout history, God has placed special people, in special places, to perform special tasks, at a special time. Never forget that God has a special place and a special task for you, too. "Not more surely is the place prepared for us in the heavenly mansions than is the special place designated on earth where we are to work for God."[1]

In the 1830's, God called a farmer out of the New England corn fields to proclaim a special message. Based on his understanding of the 2300-day prophecy in Daniel 8:14, William Miller launched a "Great Awakening," that swept across North America and Europe. The Great Disappointment that resulted when Christ did not return on October 22, 1844 as Miller had calculated He would, left thousands of his followers in bewilderment. But then God raised up individuals like James and Ellen White, Joseph Bates, Hiram Edson, J. N. Loughborough, and J. N. Andrews to form the nucleus of the Seventh-day Adventist Church. Later in the 1870's, He raised up a man to give impetus to the proclamation of a health message that was to be the "right hand" of the gospel.[2]

Vision of an Institution for Healing — It was Christmas day, 1865. Ellen White and her husband were passing through New York. They had recently left Caleb Jackson's water cure center in Dansville. Though only in his early forties, James had suffered a stroke. Some of the other leaders were also suffering health problems. So they had gone to Jackson's "Our Home on the Hillside" for recuperation. In describing the experience Ellen White said, "We had confidence in the use of water as one of God's appointed remedies, but no confidence in drugs."[3] She also wrote that she had been shown that at the time Our Home was "the best health institution in the United States."[4]

Now they were on their way back to Battle Creek and had stopped in Rochester where they had lived for three years. On this holiday, Mrs. White received her second major vision on health reform. While the vision built on the principles of healthful living that God had previously given one and a half years earlier at Otsego, Michigan, it is best remembered for its instructions for Adventists to establish their own institution in which these health principles could be taught and practiced.

J. N. Loughborough, a member of the Battle Creek, Michigan congregation was appointed fund raiser for the $11,000 project. He started contacting various members of the church but didn't have any success until he came to the broom factory of John Preston Kellogg.

In 1834, Mr. Kellogg moved his family from Massachusetts to a farm near the present city of Flint, Michigan, about 75 miles north of Detroit. Three years later, John watched as his first wife's health slowly deteriorated. Despite, or maybe because of, periodic bleeding and faithfully following the doctor's instructions to "inhale fumes of resin sprinkled over live coals" Mary met an untimely death in her teens. It is possible that Mr. Kellogg also recalled his own suffering from an eye malady. After being treated with heavy dosages of calomel, his tongue swelled so much that it protruded from his mouth and copious amounts of saliva drooled down his chin while for the next ten years he suffered bouts of chronic diarrhea.[5] No doubt he also thought of Ella, the beloved 2-year-old infant he had buried. When an autopsy proved that the worthless treatments she had been given in her illness were based on a misdiagnosis, "both parents were disgusted with the lack of medical skill of the doctor" and began subscribing to the *Water Cure Journal.*[6] Their belief in natural healing was solidified when treatments recommended therein were used to successfully treat a measles epidemic in 1850.[7]

Yes, the owner of the only broom factory between Detroit and Chicago, had experienced more than his share of blood, drugs, and tears. So he asked Mr. Loughborough how much had been raised for the proposed health institution.

"Nothing yet," was the uninspiring reply.

Kellogg straightened up. Taking the contributor's list from Loughborough's hands he signed his name boldly, and inked $500 next to it. "Understand, that this $500 is a seed to start the new institution, sink or swim."[8]

Now Kellogg worked in his broom factory from 12–14 hours a day at 75 cents a day. You do the math. In pledging $500 he had committed two years worth of salary.

Oh, and did I mention, he had sixteen children to feed!

Loughborough was so excited that he immediately ran over to the White's home to tell them of the good news. Ellen herself then pledged another $500. From these two gifts the Western Health Reform Institute, the first Adventist medical institution, had its beginnings.

Every time I read this story I am humbled. I am chastised. I am reproved for my lack of faith. How many of us have enough faith to pledge two weeks of salary to the work of God, let alone two years? I think I might have done it once — a long time ago — when the sacrifice wasn't as great as it would be now. Far too often when the offering plate is passed, I find myself digging deep into my pocket to find a crumpled dollar or two. Then I label it "benevolent giving." How sad!

When I was a child, it was customary for Adventist churches to hold an annual Week of Sacrifice. Members were encouraged to give a week's salary to start missionary work in new places. And it did something for God's people. It stretched their faith. It built their confidence in a God who could supply every necessity without the efforts of mankind. It made believers more cognizant of the need to walk by faith and not by sight.

Sabbath School investment is another program that has gone by the wayside in many churches. Here was another opportunity to put God to the test. On "Investment Sabbath," the leader would challenge members to put some small project in the hands of God and give the proceeds to His work. Then during the year, as God blessed, members shared their experiences with the rest of the church.

These were not complicated endeavors that took a lot of time and energy. No, they were simple, yet edifying.

Examples included:
• Collecting one's loose change at the end of each day and saving it in a cookie jar.
• Raising one's own produce and selling the extra crops.
• Giving a dollar for every "A" a student got on his or her report card.
• Donating the proceeds from a yard sale.

The dollar amounts were generally small; less than one hundred dollars per person. Yet how thrilling to hear the accounts of God's multiplication of man's minutia so by the time the investment period had ended, several thousand dollars had been raised to further the gospel work.

But it wasn't just in the economic arena that our pioneers sacrificed. Evangelism was their way of life. They believed Jesus was coming soon and there was a world that needed to be warned. There are accounts of Joseph Bates walking miles in the snow in the dead of winter to give a Bible study. Too often I don't have the courage to even walk next door to share my faith.

And young people were involved. Ellen White had her first vision when she was but seventeen. Her husband James had baptized hundreds by the time he was in his early twenties. I strongly suggest you read their accounts as recorded in such books as <u>Life Sketches</u> by Ellen White and <u>The Great Second Advent Movement</u> by J. N. Loughborough. The stories will thrill your soul and give you greater confidence in the God we serve.

I do not know how John Preston Kellogg managed to feed his family over the next couple of years. Yet I can find nothing in the historical record that tells of anyone in his family going hungry or without clothes. On the contrary, it seems that his business prospered.

Ellen White wrote: "... the work of God was founded in a sacrifice, and only by a sacrifice can it be carried forward."[9] May God help us to catch the vision and spirit of sacrifice of our early pioneers.

Early Days of the Western Health Reform Institute — On September 5, 1866 the Western Health Reform Institute opened its doors with a staff of two physicians, one nurse, three or four helpers, and two bath attendants. Rates ranged from five to seven dollars per week. That fee was all inclusive of room, meals, nursing care, treatments, and medical fees. Patients began coming from all over the eastern United States and Canada for the "water cures". They came in such large numbers that some had to be housed in the surrounding farmhouses as there wasn't enough room for them at the institute.

During its first 10 years of operation, it served 2000 patients. Of these ten died, an average of one per year.[10] Such a degree of success was truly remarkable. Remember this was prior to the discovery of the germ theory of disease as set forth by Robert Koch and Louis Pasteur. No one really knew what caused sicknesses; nor how to heal them. Consequently people went to hospitals to die; not to get well.

Imagine what would happen today if a hospital only lost one patient a year, or even one a month. That hospital would be in such demand it wouldn't be able to handle all those desiring treatment. Well that is exactly what happened at the Western Health Reform Institute. It quickly was cast into the national spotlight. As conditions became more and more crowded it was obvious that something must be done. Church members and stockholders began pressing for a building program to accommodate the increasing numbers.

Emergence of John Harvey Kellogg — But a few leaders, including James and Ellen White, realized that there simply were not enough physicians to serve more patients. Especially lacking were physicians who believed in the unique Adventist approach to health care. So rather than supporting a building program, the Whites urged that more physicians be trained first.

Two of John Preston Kellogg's boys (John Harvey and his older brother, Merritt, who was already a physician), the White's two boys (Edson and Willie), and a young lady, Jennie Trembley, were sent to Dr. Russell Trall's Hygieo-Therapeutic College to study rational methods of therapy. You may recall from the previous chapter that Dr. Trall was the dean of the hydrotherapy movement in America.

In sending these promising young people to Dr. Trall's College, the leadership of the Adventist Church was giving them the best opportunity to be trained in natural healing methodologies and to avoid the noxious drugs and harmful treatments that were still largely administered by the regular or allopathic physicians. This was providential as it wasn't too many years afterwards that Dr. Trall's Hygieo College, along with many other "alternative" institutions, shut down. Since its founding in 1847, the American Medical Association (AMA), which represented the traditional regular doctors of the day, had been pushing for licensure. Medicine felt threatened by the rise of alternative options such as homeopathy, herbal medicine, and the popular hydrotherapy spas. Through organized state efforts, campaigns were waged so that only AMA members would be recognized as qualified to practice medicine.

With the closure of so many non-AMA recognized institutions, Adventist leaders recognized what was happening. Though most of the water cures were sound, and many other Adventists besides the Whites had gone to them for treatments, they could see the handwriting on the wall. If the Western Health Reform Institute were to survive, it must have trained leaders who had credentials that would be accepted by the medical establishment. Thus it was that at the end of the six-month training course at the Hygieo-Therapeutic College, John Harvey Kellogg, the most promising of the five Adventist students, was encouraged to continue his medical education.

As a young lad, John watched while a friend underwent minor surgery right on the kitchen table. The sight of blood made him so sick that he decided that when he grew up he would be "anything but a doctor."[11]

By the time he was twelve, he had decided to become a teacher. Shortly thereafter, Elder White, who at the time was president of the Seventh-day Adventist Publishing Association, invited him to learn the printing trade at the Review and Herald press. Over the next four years John Harvey worked his way up from errand boy, to a typesetter, and then proofreader. Eventually he even assisted with the editorial work.

In the Review office, copies of the works of Sylvester Graham and Larkin B. Coles were for sale. In his spare time Kellogg read these. He was also exposed to the sentiments expressed in How to Live and the early issues of the *Health Reformer* while setting the type for them. Gradually he put into practice the things he learned from these publications. One of his first lifestyle changes was to adopt a vegetarian diet, despite the fact that meat was regular fare in the Kellogg home and he was especially fond of richly browned oxtails.

When he arrived at Trall's Hygieo-Therapeutic College, the younger Kellogg still had no desire to become a physician. He felt it would be worthwhile however to learn what he could about health education. Due to a lack of instructors at the college, plus his keen mind and teaching background, it wasn't long before John was asked to teach the chemistry courses.

Upon his return to Battle Creek, James White again took John under his wing. Elder White encouraged him to continue his medical training at the University of Michigan in Ann Arbor. In the early 19th century, four faculty members were considered a minimum for a medical school. A full course of instruction required attendance for two terms, each one being four–six months in duration. The second term was but a repeat of the first, as it was believed that repetition was one of the best methods of education. If at the end of the second term a student passed an exam, he received his medical degree. Clinical experience was largely obtained by being apprenticed to a practicing physician.

After his first term at Michigan, Kellogg's views regarding medicine changed. He decided to attend the best medical school possible. With a $1,000 loan from the Whites to cover his expenses, John matriculated at the Bellevue Hospital Medical School in New York, which was noted for its emphasis on combining clinical experience with classroom teaching.

On February 25, 1875, just one day before his 23rd birthday, John Harvey Kellogg graduated with an M.D. degree. One year later, he was appointed Medical Superintendent of the Western Health Reform Institute. The next year, Kellogg changed the name of the institute to Battle Creek Medical and Surgical Sanitarium, commonly known as the Battle Creek Sanitarium.

The "Sanitarium" — It was Kellogg who actually coined the word "sanitarium." At the time, *sanatoriums* were fairly widespread. A *sanatorium* was an establishment that utilized physical agents in the restorative process of the chronically ill, in particular tuberculosis patients. From its inception Battle Creek San emphasized hydrotherapy; along with diet, exercise, and other physical means of rehabilitation. But Kellogg felt "sanitarium" would place more emphasis on the concept of sanitation, or an institution where "sanitary" measures were employed to prevent the growth and spread of germs. He chose the spelling in the same year that Pasteur was presenting his germ theory of disease to the French Academy of Sciences and believed that the name, *sanitarium*, would come to mean "a place where people learn to stay well."[12] In later years Kellogg remarked that the Sanitarium was more like a "university of health" than it was a hospital.

Kellogg was proud of the fact that he got "sanitarium" into the dictionary.[13] However, getting the word into the mainstream English vocabulary was another matter, as the concept never really caught on outside of Adventism. I remember that in my childhood, most Adventist medical institutions incorporated "Sanitarium" into their names. For example, I was born in the Washington Sanitarium and Hospital. It has since been renamed Washington Adventist Hospital. In Asia, the Tokyo Sanitarium and Hospital is now called Tokyo Adventist Hospital. In the Philippines, rather than a Manila Sanitarium and Hospital, there is now a Manila Adventist Hospital. And if you were to look up the word "sanitarium" in a Webster's dictionary, much to Dr. Kellogg's chagrin, were he still alive, you would find but a one-word definition, "*sanatorium.*"

When Kellogg took over the leadership of the Institute on October 1, 1876, some of its physicians and patients showed their disapproval by leaving. Thus Kellogg began his administration with only twelve clients at the Institute. Yet under his leadership and the blessings of the Lord, within a decade, Battle Creek Sanitarium became the largest institution of its kind in the world.

The Genius of Dr. John Harvey Kellogg — It is simply amazing the talents with which Dr. John Harvey Kellogg was blessed. He was a surgeon, administrator, health reformer, nutritionist, inventor, author, and speaker. It seems incredible that all those labels could be effectively worn by one individual.

Beginning at the age of 23,[14] and continuing until he was 88, he performed over 22,000 operations.[15] At one time he set a new record by performing 162 successive abdominal surgeries without a fatality. This was at a time when 15–20% of patients undergoing abdominal surgery were expected to die.[16] Ellen White stated that it was Kellogg's dependence on divine aid that accounted for this surgical skill. She wrote that in vision she had seen a heavenly being standing at his side and guiding his hands as he operated.[17]

He spoke to hundreds of thousands of Americans in over 5,000 public lectures. He published nearly 50 books, one of them 1,680 pages in length. A number of these were written in an unbelievably short period of time. One of his early endeavors, <u>The Uses of Water in Health and Disease </u>took just eight days and he did not have the benefit of Microsoft Word. His <u>Plain Facts about Sexual Life</u> took just two weeks to write and sold over half a million copies. His most comprehensive book on nutrition was <u>The New Dietetics</u>. An editor of the *New York Evening Post* thought that it qualified Kellogg for a Nobel Prize as a "life saver."

The doctor usually wrote entirely from memory with only a brief outline of chapter headings as a guide. Oh, that all of us had such photographic memories! The story is told that he could often be seen riding his bicycle to work while a secretary ran alongside him taking down dictation.

In an age noted for the inventions of Thomas Edison, Henry Ford, and Alexander Graham Bell; Kellogg also made his contribution by patenting devices in the field of medicine. He invented or modified and improved a variety of contraptions including ones to increase blood circulation, to improve digestion, and to aid in weight loss. The vibrating belt, still used in some weight reduction salons, was his invention. In 1894 he perfected the universal dynamometer for testing grip strength. He designed another dynamometer for testing all the major muscle groups in the body. The tanning booth, menthol inhaler to clear nasal passages, the mechanical horse for exercise, and the vibrating chair were other products of his creative mind.

These, along with many other inventions are on display at the Kellogg Center in the Adventist Heritage Village on Van Buren St. in Battle Creek. At least two types of exercise equipment, the mechanical horse and his rowing machine, sunk aboard the *Titanic*, the first ocean liner to have a gym.

As a health reformer, he was a strong proponent of vegetarianism believing that not only was it unhealthy to eat meat of any kind but to do so was directly contrary to the teachings of the Bible. On one occasion, to drive home a point during a lecture at the San, he sent for a prime beefsteak from one of Battle Creek's most exclusive restaurants. He then directed a bacteriologist to examine both the steak and some barnyard manure under a microscope. The results? There was more harmful bacteria in the beefsteak than in the animal dung.

He was not afraid to lock horns with the powerful meat packing industry. Upton Sinclair in his classic novel, The Jungle, had called attention to the deplorable conditions that existed in the meat packing industry. It caused such an uproar among the American populace that in response, the United States government organized the Department of Agriculture to assure the public that meat from American cattle ranches was safe to eat. The meat industry also went on a counterattack. To assure the public of the safety of government inspected beef, they came up with a jingle called, *And He Ate Meat*.

"And He Ate Meat"[18]

Methuselah ate what he found on his plate,
And never, as people do now,
Did he note the amounts of the calorie count;
He ate it because it was chow.

He wasn't disturbed as at dinner he sat,
[Devouring] a roast or a pie,
To think it was lacking in granular fat,
Or a couple of vitamins shy.

"He cheerfully chewed every species of food,
Untroubled by worries or fears,
Lest his health might be hurt by some fancy dessert,
And he lived over nine hundred years!"

Kellogg could not take this sitting down. Since boyhood he had enjoyed writing poetry, so his response to this affront by the meat industry was a 2-part verse, a portion of which follows.

"What Methuselah ate
Was not on a plate,
For plates were not yet invented.
Being discreet,
He ate Paradise meat,
And thus old age prevented.
For Paradise meat
Was delicious to eat,
And kept him in finest condition.
And 'twas hung on trees,
And not made to please
The deadly Live Stock Commission...."

With his interest in foods and belief that vegetarianism was the healthiest diet, Kellogg promoted the development of meat analogs. In addition, he is credited with inventing two popular foods eaten today around the world; peanut butter and corn flakes.

Local folklore has it that one day while walking past the hospital kitchen, Kellogg smelled something burning. Stopping to investigate, he found the young man responsible for roasting peanuts distracted by his girlfriend and not paying attention to his job. Angry, at the neglect, Kellogg told him he would have to pay for the burnt peanuts.

Upset, the boy walked home. Once there he decided to take out his frustration on a handful of peanuts that were in his pocket. He proceeded to place them on the floor and smash them with a hammer. Rather than shattering as expected, the peanuts metamorphosed into a soft gooey mess.

He put the paste on a platter, returned to the sanitarium, and there waited outside Kellogg's office. When the doctor emerged on his way to surgery, the young man held out the paste for Kellogg to sample. Kellogg liked it and from there went on to develop peanut butter.

Administering a hospital, performing surgeries, lecturing, inventing foods and exercise equipment, writing books, plus opening his home to forty-two orphan and foster children give evidence of Kellogg's workaholic tendencies. He demanded of himself a punishing schedule and seldom got more than four hours of sleep at night. As to his diet, his own eating habits were quite irregular, even though he was careful about what he ate. Often he was so busy that he wouldn't take time to eat regular meals, preferring to snack on dried fruits and nuts as he worked.

I sympathize with him, as I too find myself struggling with these issues. Perhaps that is why I appreciate the humor in the following anecdote recorded by Richard Schwarz: *"I am under no obligation to practice what I preach. My business is to preach, and really I haven't time to practice. I am putting out fires; that is my business. I belong to the fire department, and I haven't time to look after my own health. I am looking after other people's health, and my own health has to take the best chance it can."*[19]

This tendency to neglect his own health, especially in matters of sleep and overwork, almost cost him his life on several occasions. Yet he always seemed capable of battling back. When he felt illness coming on, he would frequently escape Michigan for the more favorable climate of Florida, a habit that I have found is still promoted among Michiganders, especially during the damp, dreary winter months. After a period of recuperation, away from the hubbub of his obligations, he would return to Battle Creek and plunge back into the same unrelenting schedule until he again approached the breaking point.

His last battle came in 1943. Following a brief bout of acute bronchitis that developed into pneumonia, this man, who more than any other was responsible for bringing the Adventist health message into the limelight, passed to his death near midnight on December 14; the same day of the year on which President George Washington had died almost 150 years earlier.

About 30 years before his death, a colleague, Dr. David Paulson, recalled a conversation he had had with the sage of Battle Creek back in 1890.[20]

Kellogg: *"Do you know how Battle Creek Sanitarium was able to keep five years ahead of the medical profession?"*

Paulson: *"No, I do not."*

Kellogg: *"When something new was brought out in the medical field, I knew from my knowledge of the spirit of prophecy whether or not it belonged in our system. If it did, I instantly adopted it. While the rest of the doctors were slowly feeling their way, I had a five year head start on them.*

On the other hand, when the medical profession was caught up in some new fad, if it did not fit the light we had received, I wouldn't touch it. By the time the doctors discovered their mistake, they wondered how it was that Dr. Kellogg did not get caught."

The Scriptures say, *"Believe in the Lord your God, and you shall be established; believe His prophets and you shall prosper."* II Chronicles 20:20

More than 100 years ago, a young John Harvey Kellogg took those words to heart. As a result, within years of his becoming physician-in-chief of a small struggling Western Health Reform Institute, that facility became the largest of its kind, attracting clientele from around the world.

Yet on the morning of February 18, 1902, this monument to healthful living lay in ashes, totally gutted by fire. Unperturbed and ignoring the counsel of the prophet who had been behind his success, Dr. Kellogg rebuilt on a much grander scale as he accelerated down a slippery slope that eventually took both himself and the Battle Creek Sanitarium out of the auspices of the Seventh-day Adventist Church. As the world entered the twentieth century, Adventism was approaching some of its darkest days.

CHAPTER 7

FROM GLORY TO AGONY

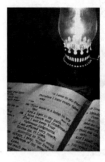

O Jerusalem, Jerusalem, the one who kills the prophet and stones those who are sent to her!

How often I wanted to gather your children together, as a hen gathers her chickens under her wings, but you were not willing!

See! Your house is left to you desolate.

Matthew 23:37, 38

April 14, 1912 — The North Atlantic Ocean, 375 miles southeast of Newfoundland, Canada — It was almost midnight. Beneath a starlit, yet moonless sky, the 890 foot long *RMS Titanic* ploughed through the ocean swells on her maiden voyage from Southhampton, England to New York. Among her 2,228 passengers and crew were some of the world's wealthiest financiers as well as the hundreds in the 3rd class compartment who had scrimped and saved every dime they had in order to sail on the "unsinkable" to begin life afresh in a "new world."

Though it was late, the parties and dances continued in her saloons and dining halls. Captain Edward J. Smith had navigated these treacherous waters for 26 years without incident. A few years earlier he had gone on record as saying, *"Of course there have been winter gales, and storms, and the like. But in all my experience, I have never been in any accident...or any sort worth speaking about. I have seen but one vessel in distress in all my years at sea. I never saw a wreck and never have been wrecked nor was I ever in any predicament that threatened to end in disaster of any sort."*[1]

Yet for some inexplicable reason,[2] Captain Smith raced full throttle through an ice field at 23 knots per hour. Nor did eight telegrams warning of the dangers ahead slow him down. Why not? Jay Henry Mowbray, one of the first to give a detailed account of the sinking puts it thus, "The captain knew, but his lips are sealed in death as, a self-inflicted bullet in his brain, he lies in the cold embrace of the sea he had loved and had defied-too long."[3]

Suddenly there was a grinding, ripping sound as below her decks, the *Titanic* was shredded from stem to engine room on the starboard side. Water quickly filled one supposedly watertight compartment after another until within a little over two hours the great behemoth slithered beneath the icy waters, taking three quarters of her passengers with her. Almost 100 years later, the sinking of the "unsinkable" *Titanic* on April 14–15, 1912, remains the greatest boat disaster in peacetime history. How eerily similar this tragedy was to a dream Ellen White had several years earlier.

"One night a scene was clearly presented before me. A vessel was upon the waters, in a heavy fog. Suddenly the lookout cried, "Iceberg just ahead!" There, towering high above the ship, was a gigantic iceberg. An authoritative voice cried out, "Meet it!" There was not a moment's hesitation. It was a time for instant action. The engineer put on full steam, and the man at the wheel steered the ship straight into the iceberg. With a crash she struck the ice. There was a fearful shock, and the iceberg broke into many pieces, falling with a noise like thunder to the deck. The passengers were violently shaken by the force of the collisions, but no lives were lost. The vessel was injured, but not beyond repair. She rebounded from the contact, trembling from stem to stern, like a living creature. Then she moved forward on her way."[4]

Adventism In Crisis — Had the *Titanic* met the iceberg head-on, its bulkhead system of watertight compartments probably would have saved the vessel from going down.[5] Interestingly enough, this dream had nothing to do with the *Titanic*. No, what Ellen White saw in vision was a threat so potentially fatal to the future of Adventism that she would refer to it as "the alpha of deadly heresies."[6] But I'm getting ahead of the story.

By the early 1900's, Battle Creek had become a metropolis of Adventist speculators. The West side of town was derogatorily deemed the "Adventist mining camp."[7] Within walking distance of the Sanitarium, near the banks of the Kalamazoo River, stood the Review and Herald publishing house. A block away the Dime Tabernacle held capacity crowds of 3,400. On Sabbath mornings, 173 separate Sabbath School classes met. Battle Creek was also home to the General Conference offices, a growing health food industry for the manufacturing and marketing of foods being developed by Kellogg, an orphanage, and a complete education system from elementary school to college.

Dwarfing everything was the sprawling Battle Creek Sanitarium complex. Stretching for a fifth of a mile along Washington Ave., it had grown to where it now employed 1000 workers. Lewis Walton in his books <u>Omega</u> and <u>Omega II</u> indicates that for many of God's people, their calling had become nothing more than "a way of making a living."[8] He goes on to graphically pen Kellogg's behind the scenes maneuvering to rewrite the Sanitarium by-laws in such a way that ownership would eventually be stripped from the church. He writes that Dr. Kellogg's sinister plan seemed innocent to all except a 72-year-old lady in far away Australia.[9]

It is baffling that Ellen White would even be in Australia at a time when the church was heading into crisis. Twelve years earlier, at the Minneapolis camp meeting in 1888, the messages preached by Alonzo T. Jones and E. J. Waggoner on righteousness by faith and the atonement, had sparked revival and reformation among Adventists.

Not since 1844 had such evangelistic fervor been manifested in the church.

Following that revival meeting, Ellen White wrote stirring counsels to church leaders. Her testimonies to ministers called for deeper consecration. Teachers were warned against adopting worldly policies. Stern instruction was given to administrators against the ongoing concentration of funds and workers in Battle Creek. In particular the publishing house and the sanitarium were in danger of losing the vision for which they had been established. Many of her direct counsels to the church at this time can be found in <u>Testimonies for the Church, Volume VI</u>.

For strong-willed men like Kellogg and some of the other church administrators, it was not easy to accept counsel and rebuke from the prophet. Even though the recipients of the testimonies, for the most part believed that Ellen White had a direct connection to heaven; it was still hard for them to accept advice that was antagonistic to their ambitions, especially since it was coming from a woman.

The burgeoning mission work provided an opportunity to surreptitiously devise a plan to send Ellen White to Australia to help advance the work there. The quickest passage was via steamship. This took several weeks. Without the modern day conveniences of telephones and the Internet, the brethren undoubtedly felt smug that at last Sister White would not be such an irritating thorn in their sides.

It was now the beginning of a new century. Mrs. White had been in Australia for almost nine years. Recently her mind could not rest. She was deeply troubled for in visions of the night she had seen strange meetings and a white-suited man with a power of persuasion unexplainable in human terms.

"Where was Dr. John Harvey Kellogg taking the Adventist medical work?" she worried. It seemed as if "the right arm of the gospel message," was being severed from the body.

Urgent words flowed from her pen to George Irwin, President of the General Conference, "Save Dr. Kellogg from himself. He is not heeding the counsel he should heed."[10]

A few days before Christmas a letter reached Dr. Kellogg's desk. "Dear Brother, I would help you if I could, but I do not know how to help you ..."[11]

And a few weeks later, "I write to you as a mother would write to her son. I would go to see you if I could.... If you receive the messages of warning given to you, it will save you from great trial and mortification, and will be the saving of your soul."[12]

To a large degree the future of the Seventh-day Adventist church was hanging in the balance. A "movement of destiny" was hurtling towards a cataclysmic turning point. Adventism was on the threshold of a day of great opportunity; it was also a day fraught with grievous danger.

The Battle Creek Sanitarium Fire — February 18, 1902 — In the frigid pre-dawn winter hours, fire gongs sounded within the Battle Creek Fire Department. Across the street, Battle Creek Sanitarium was ablaze. In less than two hours most of the edifice was nothing more than a mass of smoldering ashes. One fireman later remarked that pouring water on the flames only seemed to add to their fury.

The cause of the fire was never determined. Just as the *Titanic* was "unsinkable," so had the main sanitarium building and hospital been declared to be "fireproof." On every floor fire hoses had been connected to the main water supply and each floor had been separated from the next with fireproofing material. Along the outside of the building, fire escapes had been built in strategic locations. The male employees were organized into fire brigades and trained to fight any fires until the fire department could arrive.

But there was an Achilles' heel. Under the brick façade lay a wooden structure. The extensive network of ventilating ducts that ran through this structure to bring fresh air into patients' rooms, provided a conduit through which any conflagration could rapidly spread once it was underway.[14]

Kellogg was out of town on a business trip. Upon hearing the news of the fire from a reporter in Chicago, he spent the rest of the trip sketching plans for a bigger and better building. It was a plan that went directly against the counsel of the Spirit of Prophecy.

"It is not the Lord's will for His people to erect a mammoth sanitarium in Battle Creek or in any other place....

"Was the Battle Creek Sanitarium consumed by fire in order that the plans might be enlarged, greater buildings erected, and more display made? I think if there were more praying, more earnest study of God's ways and purposes for the advancement of his work, we would see our brethren taking a course altogether different from the course that some are now taking."[15]

One can only wonder how different Adventist history might have been, if at this critical junction, Dr. John Harvey Kellogg had put his personal pride and ambitions aside and listened to prophetic counsel. From his boyhood, Dr. Kellogg had maintained a close relationship with the Whites. You may recall from the previous chapter how as a young boy, Elder White had taken John under his wing and became a father figure to him. There was a period of time when the young John Harvey actually lived in the White's home. He had attended Trall's Hygieo-Therapeutic College with the two White boys. And it was James White who later lent him money to attend medical school.

Early in his career, Dr. Kellogg had strongly supported Ellen White's writings on health. In the *Preface* to <u>Christian Temperance and Bible Hygiene,</u> a collection of James and Ellen White's combined early writings on health he wrote, *"... the writings (herein) not only bore the stamp of truth, but were indorsed as such by a higher than human authority,"* and then went on to say, *"... At the present time, every one of the principles advocated more than a quarter of a century ago is fortified in the strongest possible manner by scientific evidence."*[16]

Yet somewhere along the way, the "genius" who admitted his professional success was due to following the counsel of Ellen White, came to the point where he felt he no longer needed to follow that counsel, if it challenged his own ambitions.

Kellogg's plans for rebuilding were costly. They far exceeded the coverage provided by the sanitarium's fire insurance policy. Alternative means of financing were necessary.

"The Alpha of Deadly Heresies" — In committee, General Conference President A. G. Daniels recalled how Ellen White had written Christ's Object Lessons with the specific purpose of raising funds for Adventist education. He wondered whether Dr. Kellogg might not follow her example and write a medical book for laymen with the proceeds going towards the rebuilding of the sanitarium. Dr. Kellogg readily agreed. The title of the book — The Living Temple.

There was only one problem. For sometime Kellogg had been formulating ideas which were very similar to concepts espoused by today's New Age movement. Subtle concepts of Eastern mysticism that depicted God as a mysterious spirit who resides everywhere in nature, found their way into the draft of The Living Temple.

Especially in the *Preface* and the first chapter of this 500 page volume, pantheistic subtleties were expressed that spiritualized away the personality and individuality of the members of the Godhead. After the book was published, Ellen White wrote that the spiritualistic theories contained therein would if "followed to their logical conclusion, sweep away the whole Christian economy."[17] Appalled, she denounced such misleading errors stealthily creeping into the church and pronounced these spiritualistic sentiments as "the alpha of deadly heresies." And she went on to say that these sentiments were so dangerously deceptive that God's people should not even explore them for the supposed purpose of being able to more effectively counteract such teachings.[18]

Meanwhile, in the editorial offices of the Review and Herald, a rather unusual event took place. The book approval reading committee decided by a vote of three to two to go ahead and publish the book. But at the 1902 Autumn Council, the decision was overturned. The minority recommendations would stand. The book would not be published.

It is at this point that one witnesses the results of what former Amazing Facts evangelist Joe Crews called "the creeping compromise." For sometime, the Review and Herald Publishing Company had been accepting outside orders. And why shouldn't they? Didn't it make good business sense to increase revenues and profit. To the despair of Mrs. White, some of those profits were coming from publications that contained sentiments contrary to Adventist teachings. Even spiritualistic publications had come off the Review's presses.

John Kellogg seized hold of the opportunity. "Print 5,000 copies of The Living Temple and charge it to the account of J.H. Kellogg," he commanded.[19]

And so the plates were set. Reams of paper were readied to receive the ink. Impervious to the deadly peril contained within its pages, the printers were ready to run the presses. Meanwhile, "in visions of the night," far away in St. Helena, California, a graying old lady, recently returned from her decade tenure in Australia, saw, "an angel standing with a sword as of fire stretched over Battle Creek."[20]

In the early evening hours of December 30, 1902, prayer meeting had just started in the Tabernacle Church. Suddenly fire alarms again clanged in the halls of the Battle Creek Fire Department. This time it was the publishing house, located on the southeast corner of West Michigan and South Washington, just a few blocks from the sanitarium grounds, that was rapidly going up in smoke. In an hour, Michigan's largest and most modern publishing house was nothing more than a pile of smoldering bricks and melted presses. Somewhere in the ruins lay the glowing embers of <u>The Living Temple</u>.

The Rebuilt Sanitarium — Magnificence and Opulence Personified — Undaunted, Kellogg went to an outside press and got his book published. With its proceeds, the doctor embarked on a rebuilding campaign that culminated in Battle Creek Sanitarium achieving a scale of magnificence and opulence, rarely seen in America at the time. The main building reflected an imposing Italian Renaissance design. It was nearly a fifth of a mile long and six stories high. A gymnasium and two flanking treatment rooms extended from the rear of the building. Its central rotunda housed a garden with parrots and butterflies flitting amongst fig, banana, orange, and palm trees. Patients walking from the main hospital building to the gym had to pass through this tropical paradise.[21]

Surrounding the hospital were 32,000 square feet of porches and verandas on which patients could take in the fresh air and sunlight, so vital to Kellogg's treatment regimen. To insulate against a repeat conflagration, each floor of the building was built with reinforced concrete. Further fire protection was afforded by the nearly five acres of marble mosaic laid down on top of the concrete. Pillars and beams were made of iron and cement. According to the *Battle Creek Idea* of May 1904 it was "the only absolutely fire-proof institution of the sort in the world."[22]

Though even before this elaborate structure was built, Battle Creek's healing qualities were known worldwide, its new grandeur along with affiliated institutions, seemed to attract the rich and the famous. In Richard Schaeffer's book <u>Legacy</u>, a Who's Who of patients and guests is provided.[23] The list includes auto magnates Henry Ford and James Buick, financier John D. Rockefeller, Edgar Welch of grape juice fame, department chain store founders J.C. Penny and Montgomery Ward, playwright George Bernard Shaw, author and motivational speaker Dale Carnegie, tennis champion Bill Tilden, Olympic swimmer

Johnny Weismuller, politician William Jennings Bryan, scientist Ivan Pavlov, Frederick Grant Banting (discover of insulin), brothers Charles and William Mayo, founders of the famous Mayo Clinic, inventor Thomas Edison, polar explorer Admiral Richard Byrd, civil rights advocate Booker T. Washington, Civil War nurse and founder of the American Red Cross, Clara Barton, and aviator Amelia Earhart.

The 23rd president of the United States, William Howard Taft, was given a complete physical examination as patient number 100,000. Amelia Earhart once gave Kellogg an aerial tour of the city of Battle Creek and its famous hospital grounds. Olympian Johnny Weismuller broke his own swimming record after he became a vegetarian under Dr. Kellogg's guidance. He later gained additional notoriety as a *Tarzan* movie actor. On the night the sanitarium burned down, one of the guests was Ira Sankey, noted hymn writer, singing evangelist, and longtime associate of Dwight L. Moody.[24]

Battle Creek Sanitarium had been the epitome of health care in the United States and Kellogg intended to keep it that way. To him, the fire had provided an opportunity to rectify problems associated with having limited space. A scaled down rebuilding program did not fit into his grandiose vision for health care in America. He was not about to let some "ignorant" ministers or a graying woman in California dictate to him Battle Creek Sanitarium's future.

Kellogg Separates From Adventism — Even before the fire though, Kellogg had found it increasingly difficult to work with church leadership. As time went on he even became critical of Ellen White, often rejecting her personal counsel to him on the basis that "she had been misinformed." He certainly was at odds with her in his plans to rebuild the Battle Creek Sanitarium. Ellen White had repeatedly urged that the hospital be kept on a small scale and that institutions in many places should be established rather than concentrating all the personal and resources in Battle Creek.

As time went on Kellogg grew increasingly bitter and antagonistic. He felt that some in church leadership were deliberately trying to break him down. Richard Scwhartz states that on at least three separate occasions serious efforts were made to heal the wounds and to bring about reconciliation. The last serious attempt took place in Berrien Springs in 1904. "W. C. White later reported that his mother firmly believed that Dr. Kellogg would have been permanently saved for the Adventist cause if some of his associates had only encouraged him to humble himself and strive once more for harmony with the ministry."[25]

On October 7, 1907, Elder Augustin C. Bordeau and George C. Amadon, members of the Battle Creek Tabernacle met for seven hours in Kellogg's home to try to ascertain what his true theological beliefs were and his attitudes towards the Spirit of Prophecy. Since Kellogg had been suspicious of the church for some time, he had stenographers take down extensive notes on what was said in any meetings with church officials. J. T. Case and Mr. Ashley recorded what transpired at that early fall meeting.[26]

During their time together, Kellogg did his best to clear his name of any wrong doing. He avowed that he was not a pantheist, that he had sought to work with church leadership to remove anything that was objectionable from The Living Temple, that he still believed in and taught the same truths of Seventh-day Adventism that he had held for more than forty years, and that he had sought to manage the Sanitarium with the utmost integrity, and to teach and live the principles of health reform.

He also indicated his belief that his "enemies" were out to destroy him and that he believed there was a concerted effort to have his name removed from church membership. *"As far as my connection with the church is concerned I expect to be turned out by the church, but I shall make no protest against it. I will not on any account withdraw from the church, and I will not ask to have my name dropped; I will do nothing of the kind, because if I do, that will immediately be used as a pretense and published everywhere that I have withdrawn from the church...*

I believe just what I have believed for the last forty years, and I am standing by everything I have stood by. I have not changed. The Conference has changed its attitude towards me and toward this institution for campaign purposes and for the purpose of subjugating us... I believe the general principles of the Seventh-day Adventist faith as it has been taught and I was taught."[27]

Just thirty-four days after this interview, Dr. John Harvey Kellogg was officially removed from church membership by the Battle Creek Tabernacle congregation, even though he wasn't present at the meeting to defend himself

Dr. Kellogg continued to practice medicine for many more years. But never again would he know the same glory that was his while listening to the prophetic voice of Ellen White.

In 1928, another expansion project was completed. With the construction of two 15-story "Towers" facing Champion Street, the San became Battle Creek's first skyscraper. The new addition helped the Sanitarium take its place among the world's most opulent buildings, able to accommodate 1,250 guests, with a staff of 1,800.[28] Descriptive adjectives

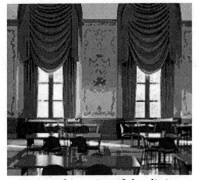

Restored interior of the dining room at the world famous Battle Creek Sanatarium.

included "hotel-like guest rooms, plush interior features, luxurious lobby with walls of the finest marble, intricately decorated ceiling, exquisite draperies and fine oriental rugs." It was opulence personified.[29]

The originally ascetic San had become quite plush,"[30] is indeed an understatement. The next year, with most of the $3 million price tag still needing to be paid, the Great Depression of 1929 struck. In 1933, Kellogg gave up the financial struggle and saw his glorious dream end in the nightmare of bankruptcy.

Today, the once mighty Battle Creek Sanitarium and Hospital still towers above the landscape of Battle Creek. It's function? A Federal Center of the United States government with its largest operation being the Defense Logistics Information Service. It also plays a key role in processing and storing information related to the Department of Homeland Security.

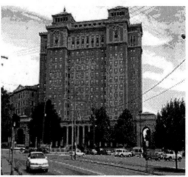

The twin towers of the former Battle Creek Sanitarium as they appear today.

On its front lawn, underneath the spreading branches of deciduous trees dating from its days of glory, a historical marker tells briefly of its former fame. Gazing past the sign towards the Corinthian colonnades supporting the portico of the Towers, one cannot help but to stand in awe and wonder "What might have been!"

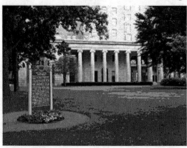

Signboard on the front lawn describing the San's former glory.

Ellen White herself posed the same thought in Testimonies Volume 8. The chapter following "The Review and Herald Fire," was addressed to the Battle Creek Tabernacle Church, and is entitled, "What Might Have Been." In vision she saw that a spirit of confession and forgiveness spread through the Battle Creek congregation. With tears and deep sorrow wrongs were made right and there was "rejoicing such as never before had been heard in the Tabernacle."

She then concludes with this distressing thought. *"I thought of where we might have been had thorough work been done at the last General Conference, and an agony of disappointment came over me as I realized that what I had witnessed was not a reality."*[31]

Out of the ashes of destruction, God's remnant people would be scattered to new destinations where other sanitariums were established. Rather than throwing monies into just one community, funds became available to start new work in many places of the world.

Today, the Seventh-day Adventist medical missionary work literally surrounds the globe with 166 hospitals and an additional 395 clinics and dispensaries operating in approximately 200 countries.[32] Sadly enough, Adventism's last medical presence in the city where it all began, the Battle Creek Lifestyle Health Center, closed its doors in 2004.

And what about Dr. Kellogg himself? At the age of ninety-one, after an acute bout of bronchitis that developed into pneumonia, he passed away on the night of December 14, 1943.

Despite turning his back on the faith which he once held dear, is it possible that Dr. John Harvey Kellogg will be in heaven? I hope so. As a public health professional, there is much about Kellogg's work and teachings that I respect and admire. Certainly the Seventh-day Adventist medical work would have never become what it was at the turn of the twentieth century, as well as what it is today, had it not been for this man that God called forth at a special time, to fill a special place in the rise of Seventh-day Adventism.

Lewis Walton provides some anecdotal data that gives me hope of someday being able to converse with Dr. Kellogg in the earth made new. Dr. Harry Miller (see chapter 10), after receiving his medical education under Kellogg, spent the greater part of his professional career in mission service to Asia. Once, while on furlough, he ran into his former professor.

Evidently, Miller had recently been reprimanded by some of the brethren. Kellogg gave him the following advice, "...don't rebel; and whatever you do, never leave the church....And don't give up on the Spirit of Prophecy."[33]

Another physician recalls how many years after Kellogg left the church he happened to meet the doctor in the dining room of an Adventist hospital. Putting his hand on the physician's shoulder he said, "Dr. Kellogg, won't you come with us?"

After a long thoughtful moment, John Harvey reportedly replied, "Perhaps, I am not as far from you as you think."[34]

CHAPTER 8

OUT OF THE ASHES

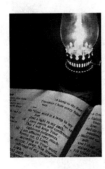

Now faith is the substance of things hoped for, the evidence of things not seen.

Hebrews 11:1

July 1905 — Los Angeles, California — Delegates from Southern California churches were meeting in emergency session. A $5,000 payment was due to secure property on which they had already placed a down payment. Not only didn't they have the $5000, they didn't even have one dollar of it. Creditors were knocking on the door, ready to foreclose. Without a miracle, the church would lose both the property and any monies invested in it up to this point.

In 1902, the same very same year that both the Battle Creek Sanitarium and Review and Herald burned down, Ellen White was shown that unoccupied properties, suitable for sanitarium work, would become available at prices far below the original costs.[1] In 1904, Paradise Valley near San Diego was worth $25,000. It was offered to the church for $12,000. The final purchase price was $4,000.

Shortly thereafter, in Glendale, just north of Los Angeles, a $50,000 investment was made available for $26,000. Once again the settlement price was remarkably cheap — $12,000.

In another vision in the fall of 1903, Ellen White saw a sanitarium in the midst of beautiful grounds somewhere in southern California. Though no place which she had previously visited met the description of what she had seen, she mailed a letter to the brethren attending campmeeting in Los Angeles, describing the property in detail.

John Burden, manager of the St. Helena Sanitarium, was given responsibility for locating the dreamed of property. In March 1904, Elder Burden found 76 acres located sixty miles east of Los Angeles

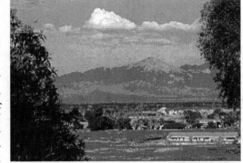

Panoramic view of the San Bernardino Valley from atop "the hill beautiful."

which met Ellen White's description. It was in the midst of a triangle formed by Riverside to the south, San Bernardino to the north, and Redlands to the east.

The 1880's had been a period of western expansion in the United States. Ever since the start of the gold rush in 1849, California had been a magnet attracting droves of people, especially to the southern region with its mild winters and dry climate. Located as it was in close proximity to the three major towns mentioned above, Loma Linda seemed to be an ideal spot for a resort.

In Spanish, *Loma Linda* means "the hill beautiful." Despite the name, the "hill" is nothing more than a small mound rising above the San Bernardino Valley. Here in the midst of citrus groves, speculators had invested in a resort that went bankrupt. A group of physicians then spent additional monies in new buildings and redecorating as they tried to turn it into a health spa. But their efforts also failed. Burden learned that he could purchase the abandoned property which was valued at $155,00 for a discounted price of $110,000.

One hundred and ten thousand dollars was a fantastic price considering what the property was worth. Yet for a church that was already burdened with paying off the debts on two other recently opened hospitals, it was out of the question. Burden left without even making a counteroffer.

Mrs. White urged Burden to return. In the interim the asking price was lowered to $85,000. But this too was out of the question. So he left again.

Mrs. White pressed him to go back a third time. This time he asked the owners for the absolute bottom line. "Forty thousand dollars, which included $15,000 worth of equipment."

This was still a high price to ask of the 1400 Seventh-day Adventists in southern California, but at least it seemed workable. The terms were $5,000 down; with equal amounts during the next three months. The remaining $20,000 would be paid at the end of three years. The lawyers came late Friday afternoon, May 26, 1905 to sign the papers. Because it was so close to the beginning of the Sabbath, Burden asked that the signing be postponed until Monday.

That weekend, Burden received a telegram from G.W. Reaser, president of the Southern California Conference. "Developments here warrant advising do not make deposit on sanitarium."

Now Burden had a dilemma. It was the kind of situation that often confronts us in our Christian walk. Would he listen to the voice of the prophet, or would he follow the wisdom of learned men who offered contrary advice.

With Mrs. White's assurance that the Lord would provide, Burden borrowed $1,000 on his own bank account to secure an option to buy the Loma Linda property.

Two weeks later, Mrs. White came to Loma Linda for the first time. As she was taken on a tour of the "Hill Beautiful," she recognized it as the very place she had been shown in vision nearly two years earlier.

Encouraged by Burden's example, local Adventists raised the additional $4,000 needed for the down payment. No one had any idea where they would get the next $5,000 that was due the following month.

And now on this warm summer day in July, time had run out. If the $5,000 payment wasn't made, the bank would foreclose on the property. The tension in the air was thick. Ellen White had said that money would come from unexpected sources. Wherever that money was, it needed to appear quickly. In the deepening desperation in the room, Elder Burden clung by faith to the assurance given by God's prophet.

Someone suggested they wait until the morning mail came. A short while later the postman arrived. In the mail was an envelope addressed from Atlantic City, New Jersey, some three thousand miles (4,800 km) away; on the other side of the United States. Nobody on the committee recognized the name of the woman on the return address. The postmark indicated that the letter had been posted weeks earlier. Inside the envelope was a bank draft for $5,000 and a letter explaining that the money was to be used in whatever way the church deemed necessary.

Yes friends, you and I have nothing to fear for the future except as we shall forget...

A man who had been critical of Burden came up to him and said, "It seems that the Lord is in this matter."

Burden replied, "He surely is and he will carry it through to victory."

No wonder the first chapel on the campus of Loma Linda University was named Burden Hall as a perpetual memorial to this mighty pillar of faith.

From that point onward, unexpected funds came flowing in from various places enabling the church to pay off the entire debt in less than six months time, saving an additional $1,100. The final cost on property valued at $155,000 was $38,900.

But the testing period was not yet over. In November of 1905, the Loma Linda Sanitarium along with a School of Nursing opened with 35 employees. Soon they learned that patient revenue was not sufficient to meet the payroll. With strong faith in the ability of God to provide, they cheerfully offered to work for only room and board until the patronage increased. That entire winter there were only 40 patients. But by June 30, 1906, sanitarium accounts were over $1,000 in the black. That same year, Ellen White emphasized, "A school is to be established here for the training of gospel medical missionary evangelists."[2]

The College of Medical Evangelists (CME), forerunner of Loma Linda University, was chartered in 1909. The timing could not have been worse. Medical education in America was in a sorry state of affairs. Only sixteen out of more than 100 recognized medical schools required even as much as two years of college education for admission. Fifty required only a high school education.

The Flexner Report Closes Medical Schools — For years the American Medical Association (AMA) had recognized that reforms were needed. There was a growing demand for medical schools to have high standards in the classrooms and adequately equipped labs. They needed to be affiliated with hospitals for clinical training.

In 1910, a report financed by the Carnegie Institute and conducted by a respected educator, Abraham Flexner, literally blasted scores of inadequately equipped medical schools out of existence. The Flexner Report was scathing in its rebuke of sub-standard institutions that were attempting to train medical practitioners. In its aftermath nearly half of the medical schools in the United States were closed down. Many of the schools of homeopathy, eclectic medicine, and osteopathy were also declared to be "hopeless" or "worthless." The College of Medical Evangelists' administrators were told it was virtually impossible for a newly established church-related medical school to measure up to the stricter standards the AMA was establishing.

Around the time of the publication of the Flexner Report, Elder Arthur G. Daniels, President of the General Conference and Homer Salisbury, Educational Secretary, were on their way from Washington D.C. to Loma

Linda for the incorporation meetings. They decided to stop in Chicago to see Dr. Nathan Colwell, Secretary of the AMA Council on Medical Education. Dr. Colwell had been given the responsibility of enforcing the new American Medical Association requirements. Elders Daniels and Salisbury wanted to get a feel for what would be necessary to have a school that met the expected standards.

They never mentioned that they were connected to Loma Linda. Yet as they rose to leave after their visit, Dr. Colwell abruptly said, "And you tell those people at Loma Linda..."

Daniels was dumbfounded that his guise hadn't worked. "And what makes you think we are from Loma Linda?" he shot back.

Colwell replied curtly, "Because no one but you Adventists think you can put on a medical school and maintain it without money."

Two years later Colwell visited the College of Medical Evangelists, evidently to close it down. Colwell didn't want any more of what he considered to be "one horse medical schools." With the Flexner Report in hand, he met with John Burden, who by this time had been appointed the institution's business manager. Burden explained to him the financial structure and mission of the Seventh-day Adventist Church. He emphasized the unique educational concept of equipping young men and women physically, mentally, and spiritually to serve humanity, not just in America, but throughout the world. Burden then made a plea to Colwell. That even though it was small and struggling, would he not take into consideration that The College of Medical Evangelists was the only school available for training workers for the unique mission of the Adventist Church.

Colwell drew solemn. "Mr. Burden, when I took my medical course, it was to become a medical missionary. The medical got me and the mission lost out."[3]

From that day forward, Dr. Nathan P. Colwell was one of the staunchest supporters of the College of Medical Evangelists. In November 1922, the School of Medicine of the College of Medical Evangelists was given an "A" rating, the highest of all rankings given by the American Medical Association.

The Legacy of Loma Linda University — Today, I believe that the greatest legacy of Loma Linda University's School of Medicine is that it has graduated more medical mission-ary physicians than

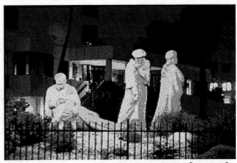

The Good Samaritan statuary in front of the School of Dentistry

any other school of medicine in the world.[4] It is a legacy that Adventists can be justly proud of. In addition to the School of Medicine, Loma Linda University now operates Schools of Public Health, Nursing, Allied Health Professions, Dentistry, and a Graduate School.

The Medical Center is the main trauma center for almost one quarter of the state of California. Approximately one third of its patients are intensive care patients. Its neonatal program, infant heart transplant program, and cancer center are world renown. Over 60% of its patients are referred from outside a 20-mile radius, this in a region teeming with very good medical facilities.

As I write this volume, Loma Linda University is celebrating its one hundredth anniversary. It is a far cry from what it was back at the turn of the twentieth century. Gone are the orange and grapefruit groves. In their place stand townhouses and condominiums as Loma Linda has become a small city in its own right. The former hospital on the hill, now known as Nichol Hall, serves the Schools of Public Health and Allied Health Professions. Meanwhile, the medical center has been relocated on several acres to the southwest of the original buildings. Even the old water tower atop the "mound" and seen in earlier pictures, has been removed.

The only trains that pass by the university's northern borders are the occasional freight trains. Gone are the rails that brought patients almost to the doorsteps of the original hospital. In their place, less than two miles away, runs the I-10 Interstate freeway which transverses the southern United States all the way from Los Angeles to Florida. A few minutes to the west, another major thoroughfare runs north and south. A bit farther away, Ontario International Airport, one of the fastest growing airports in North America, makes Loma Linda readily accessible from almost anyplace in the world.

Thus a $155,000 piece of property, that was abandoned because it had difficulty attracting people, now has become the very hub of the fastest growing area in southern California. Yet despite all the changes of the past century, one constant remains. The academic halls and classrooms are still hallowed by dedicated Christian professors who feel called by God to continue molding workers for the global mission of the Seventh-day Adventist Church.

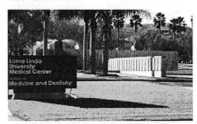

Signboard at the entrance to Loma Linda University Medical Center.

I am proud to be part of the ongoing miracle that is Loma Linda. Growing ip in a lower-middle class suburb north of Philadelphia, Pennsylvania, I never dreamed that one day I would receive advanced degrees from that institution. Financially, it was totally out of the question. Academically, it was a challenge. Yet, God made the impossible, plausible.

My wife, Mieko, is also a graduate of that great institution. And it was within the walls of the neo-natal unit that Keiko, our daughter made her entrance upon planet Earth.

I am thankful for the opportunities that were ours during the fourteen years we spent living in Loma Linda. I am also thankful for the John Burdens of the church who were willing to believe the words of the prophet and "Go Forward," when so many, even among church leadership hesitated and doubted.

"Properties would become available at far below their original cost."
E. G. W. 1903

	Value	Offered	Purchase Price
1904 - Paradise Valley	$25,000	$12,000	$4,000
1904 - Glendale	$50,000	$26,000	$12,000
1905 - Loma Linda	$155,000	$110,000	$38,900
TOTAL	$230,000	$148,000	$54,900

"The Lord still wants His people to believe that He is willing and able do just as great things for them as He did for the children of Israel in their journey from Egypt to Canaan. We are to have an educated faith that will not hesitate to follow His instructions in the most difficult experiences. "Go forward" is the command of God to His people.

"*Faith and cheerful obedience are needed to bring the Lord's designs to pass. When He points out the necessity of establishing the work in places where it will have influence, the people are to walk and work by faith. By their godly conversation, their humility, their prayers and earnest efforts, they should strive to bring the people to appreciate the good work that the Lord has established among them. It was the Lord's purpose that the Loma Linda Sanitarium should become the property of our people, and He brought* _it about at a time when the rivers of difficulty were full and overflowing their banks."_ (emphasis mine)[5]

In retrospect it can be seen that God used the conflagrations in Battle Creek to scatter His people. As a result the missionary zeal of the church was heightened. And the world began to take note. Before the 20th century came to an end, the lifestyle teachings of Adventists would be catapulted to the forefront of scientific research in such a way that Seventh-day Adventism would become synonymous with health promotion and disease prevention. And Loma Linda University Medical Center would become much more than what the pioneers of Adventism could have ever hoped or dreamed.

CHAPTER 9

"I WILL MAKE YOU THE HEAD"

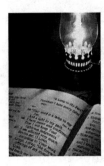

Now it shall come to pass, if you diligently obey the voice of the Lord your God, to observe carefully all His commandments which I command you today, that the Lord your God will set you high above all nations of the earth....

And the Lord will make you the head and not the tail; you shall be above only, and not be beneath, if you heed the commandments of the Lord your God, which I command you today, and are careful to observe them.

Deuteronomy 28:1, 13

December 1953 — New York City — Ernst Wynder, a young researcher at Sloan Kettering Institute of Cancer Research had just made an important discovery. He had shaved the hair off the backs of some mice and painted the bare skin with a solution containing tobacco tar. Now he noticed that skin cancers had developed in those areas in contact with the tobacco tar.[1]

The story made the nightly news as it was the first scientific experiment to definitively link tobacco with cancer. Dr. Wynder now wondered, "Could it be that tobacco smoke was responsible for the rising death toll in lung cancer that had been occurring in American men since World War II?"

To answer the question he needed two sets of people; smokers and non-smokers. Finding smokers wasn't a problem. They were all around him as about 45% of American men smoked in the 1950's. But where could he find a comparable group of average Americans who didn't smoke?

Someone on his research team suggested Seventh-day Adventists. Dr. Wynder had never heard of them. Learning that their headquarters were in Washington D. C., he placed a phone call there. They directed him to Loma Linda University's College of Medical Evange-lists. A research project was begun comparing Califor-nian Seventh-day Adventists with other Californians who were smokers. The results, published in 1964 in the pres-tigious medical journal, *Cancer*,[2] showed that Adventists had only a third of the deaths from lung cancer as did the general population. And among those who had never smoked it was extremely rare.

That initial study led to additional scientific studies evaluating the lifestyles of Seventh-day Adventists. The results have been published in various medical journals around the world. Listed on the Loma Linda University website is a link from which one can download referenc-es and abstracts for these reports, which now total more than three hundred.[3]

Between 1958 and 1965 almost 50,000 California Seventh-day Adventists were enrolled in a study pertain-ing to mortality, or causes of death. The researchers were interested in finding out if the Adventist lifestyle made any quantifiable difference in terms of longevity. It was known that most Adventists do not smoke or drink al-cohol. In addition many members were vegetarians and also abstained from the free use of caffeinated beverages, irritating spices and refined foods. Other healthful prac-tices included regular exercise, an abundant use of water combined with plenty of fresh air and sunshine. All of these practices had been emphasized since the days of Dr. Kellogg and the Battle Creek Sanitarium. But there was no published data verifying that such a lifestyle could indeed delay the inevitable day of dying.

The results of the Adventist Mortality Study showed that Adventists were reaping significant benefits from their health behaviors. Using the non-SDA Californians as a point of reference, the results showed that for many major illnesses, Adventists' death rates were far less than expected. For example, for every 100 Californians dying from lung cancer, only 20 Adventists died. For oral cancers the results were even more astounding, just five out of the expected 100. Other cancers ranged between a low of 28% of the norm for bladder cancer and a high of 72% for breast cancer. Rates for suicide, ulcers, diabetes, stroke, bronchitis, and motor vehicle accidents were also lower than the general population. Mortality from all causes was only 59% of expected numbers. In other words, for every 100 Californians dying within any comparable group, only 59 Seventh-day Adventists died.[4]

The results of the early studies indicated that at age 35, Seventh-day Adventist women could expect to live three years longer than their non-SDA counterparts, while for SDA men the Adventist advantage was an amazing six years.[5] To give an idea of the significance of this, over the last fifteen years, life expectancy at birth in the United States, has increased by less than three years. This despite the fact that since 1990, there has been a tremendous increase in medical knowledge and technology.

The noted differences were especially significant in terms of heart disease. At the time the study was conducted, heart disease was the number one killer of males between the ages of 35 and 64, who were living in the United States. But within this age group, Seventh-day Adventists males had one quarter the death rate of other Californians.[6] However, as low as this was it was still higher than among Japanese living in Japan.

Back in the 1960's Japan had one of the lowest coronary heart disease death rates in the world. Many believed that this was because the Japanese had some hereditary or genetic characteristic that protected them. Over the last 40 years this hypothesis has been soundly refuted. Today coronary heart disease and cancer are the top killers in Japan,[7] having even surpassed strokes, which for many years had held the dubious position of being number one.

By importing the American fast food diet, the Japanese are paying a high price. A number of years ago I took a walk around a segment Tokyo's business and entertainment center known as Shinjuku. Along a square kilometer perimeter I found four McDonald's, a couple of Wendy's, several donut shops, two or three ice cream parlors, and several pizza establishments. Despite the close proximity of competitors, each was doing a brisk business.

Similar scenes can be witnessed throughout Asia. In the Kowloon Peninsula of Hong Kong, within a fifteen minute walk I again encountered no less than four McDonald's, including one that is open 24-hours a day. As Orientals seek to eat like Americans, they have started to die like Americans. In most Asian countries, the top three killers are heart disease, cancer, and stroke, just like in America.

Yet, even back in the sixties, when heart disease was extremely low in Japan, Loma Linda researchers discovered that if they divided Seventh-day Adventists into vegetarians and non-vegetarians, the vegetarian Adventist males had heart disease death rates that were even lower than those of Japanese living in Japan.[8]

For more than 40 years, research on the lifestyle of Seventh-day Adventists has continued. Most of the work in the United States has been funded by the National Institutes of Health, a medical research arm of the US government. But studies have not been limited to the United States. Seventh-day Adventists living in Australia, the Netherlands, Norway, Denmark, Japan, New Zealand, Poland, Finland, and the Caribbean have been critically researched. The results are consistent — wherever the health teachings of the Seventh-day Adventist Church are practiced; death and disease decrease, and both the quantity and quality of life increases.

In 1981,[9] Norwegian researchers reported that Adventist men in their country had a four-year additional life advantage and that for women there was a two-year increased life expectancy. This difference was perceived as being equal to the "additional life which the Norwegian population would have had if ischemic heart disease had been eliminated as a cause of death."

The report stated that the "Adventist Advantage" was not due to education, economic state, genetics, or environment. In fact, Adventists tended to be at a disadvantage in these areas. They had less formal education, were in a lower economic bracket, and lived in less healthful environments. The conclusion was that it was their lifestyle, coupled with a strong religious faith, that made the health difference.

The investigators concluded their report published in the *Journal of the Norwegian Medical Association*, by saying "Health...is a function of lifestyle, and lifestyle can be chosen."[10]

Let me remind you once again of the challenge that Moses gave to Israel in his farewell address. *"I have set before you life and death, blessing and cursing: therefore choose life, that both you and your descendants may live: that you may love the Lord your God, and you may obey His voice, and that you may cling to Him, for He is your life, and the length of your days."* Deuteronomy 30:19, 20.

God is faithful to His promises. Adventists have discovered that adherence to His lifestyle principles, gives them a health advantage. At one time, Dr. T. Hirayama was the leading cancer epidemiologist in Japan. In 1981 he published the first major study establishing a link between premature death and environmental tobacco smoke or passive smoking.[11] Five years later, in 1985 he published the first scientific study of Japanese Adventists.[12] The results were so significant that he coined the term "*SDA gata*". *SDA gata* or "Seventh-day Adventist lifestyle" became a household term in Japan. People still use it to describe a total health promoting lifestyle.

A Providential Meeting — In 1986, as part of my graduate studies, I did a 10-week internship at Tokyo Adventist Hospital. While there I conducted research for my doctoral monograph. A few years earlier, Dr. Albert Bandura at Stanford University had developed a health education concept known as "self-efficacy theory." It was a model designed to predict how successful a person might be in changing a particular behavior, such as quitting smoking.

Dr. Ed Fujimoto, the Director of Health Promotion at the hospital, suggested I use participants in the hospital's stop smoking programs to test whether this theory was as valid with Asian populations as it had been among Americans. Dr. Fujimoto and I developed a questionnaire to evaluate how confident smokers were that they could refrain from smoking in a variety of situations. According to self-efficacy theory, the answers to such questionnaires should enable health educators to accurately predict those who will be successful and conversely those who will not be successful in quitting smoking over the long term. Such information is extremely valuable because it enables one to design specific interventions for those individuals who are most likely to resume smoking. In so doing the number of relapsers, can be greatly reduced.

For my monograph, I needed to include data that was current. I had no trouble finding up-to-date statistics on smoking in America. However, for Japan, I couldn't find any data that was more recent than 10-years-old. For purposes of doctoral research, such data was about as reliable as if it had been 100-years-old.

One day while browsing the bookshelves in Dr. Fujimoto's office, I noticed a publication containing proceedings from a smoking and health conference that had been held in Nagoya a few years earlier. Since my wife is from Nagoya and her family was still living there, I began to formulate a plan.

I decided to take a few days off to visit my in-laws. While there I planned to visit with Dr. Ogawa, the principle compiler of the proceedings. I mailed a letter to him explaining my need and requesting an interview.

A few days before I left for Nagoya, I got a negative reply. Dr. Ogawa would be out of town at the time of my visit. "But," he suggested, "Perhaps Dr. Tominaga, his colleague and director of cancer epidemiology at the Aichi Prefecture Cancer Center would be willing to answer my questions."

In most Oriental cultures, it is impossible to visit a man of Dr. Tominaga's stature without having an appointment. Initial appointments are usually made through an intermediary third-party, not directly. I could use Dr. Ogawa as a referral but it was too close to my departure time to arrange a visit with his colleague. My only chance was in an unannounced visit. I hoped that Dr. Tominaga would waive protocol and not feel insulted by my unexpected demands on his time.

Following my father-in-law's directions, it took about an hour and a half on public transportation for me to arrive at the Aichi Cancer Center. Standing in front of the sprawling complex, I became deeply concerned as to how I would ever find Dr. Tominaga, that is if he were even there. And if he were, would he be willing to see me?

Complicating the matter was my extremely limited Japanese language ability. Barely knowing enough to get myself into trouble, who was I to have the audacity to even think that I could get an audience with Dr. Tominaga myself. I knew that if I ran into any difficulties, my Japanese ability would be hopeless in trying to extricate myself.

As I neared the building and witnessed the hordes moving in and out, I silently prayed. At the receptionist's desk I asked in my broken Japanese, *"Eigo o hanasu no hito ga, imasu ka?"* "Does anyone here speak English?"

I was politely told to "Wait a moment." At least someone had understood my question.

Soon a young lady came to my assistance. Within moments I realized I was in serious trouble. It was hard for me to discern which was worse; my Japanese (which was just a notch above horrendous), or her English. Somehow I was able to communicate that I wanted to see Dr. Tominaga. We went down one corridor, then another. Finally stopping outside an examination room, I was told Dr. Tominaga would see me shortly.

Much to my consternation, Dr. Tominaga spoke even less English than my "translator." However, since all college educated individuals in Japan spend several years studying English, I knew that he must be fairly literate in his ability to read and write English. So I asked him if he would be willing to respond to a written set of questions if I were to send them to him.

About this time, my Japanese "friends" began figuring out the purpose of my visit.. There were several Dr. Tominagas working in the Aichi Cancer Center. I had been taken to a specialist on the clinical ward. This was not the Dr. Tominaga that I was interested in. That Dr. Tominaga worked in the research department in the basement.

Once again my guide led me along some corridors, down a cold concrete stairway, finally depositing me outside a door with the now almost expected words, "Please, wait a moment."

Time for another prayer. I had already been at the cancer center for thirty minutes and was getting frustrated with the lack of progress in finding Dr. Tominaga.

Within moments a gentleman stepped out of an office and in perfect English asked, "How can I help you?"

"I'm looking for Dr. Tominaga," I replied, relieved that at last here was someone with whom I could perhaps communicate.

"I'm Dr. Tominaga. Won't you come into my office," he offered.

I then apologized for my rudeness in coming without an appropriate appointment and began to explain the purpose of my visit, — how I was a graduate student from Loma Linda University doing research on smoking among Japanese and was trying to find data on smoking related illnesses in Japan. Not sure if he had even heard of Loma Linda, I began to explain a little bit about the institution.

Dr. Tominaga interrupted me, "I know Loma Linda University very well. Dr. Roland Phillips and I are good friends. We were graduate students together at Johns Hopkins University."

I about fell off my chair I was so astonished. At the time, Dr. Roland Phillips was the principle investigator for the Adventist Health Study. My wife was working for him as a computer programmer.

I ended up spending two hours in Dr. Tominaga's office. During our visit he volunteered, "Next month I am to present a paper in Russia on *Smoking and Disease in Japan*. I have just finished compiling the data for it. This data shows morbidity and mortality data for smoking related illnesses in Japan. The figures are so recent that they haven't even been published yet. I will share this data with you if you will give me your word that they will not appear anywhere in print before the end of September."

This was the exact data that I needed for my research. Data so new that even the average Japanese didn't have access to it yet!

When I returned that evening to the home of my non-Christian in-laws they could hardly believe my story. They concluded that indeed a miracle had happened.

Years later, after serving a combined nine years in Hong Kong and the Philippines, I decided that my family and I needed to return to the States for a period of time. As I browsed several job search engines on the Internet, I was intrigued by a university in Michigan that was starting a new Bachelor's program in "Wellness, Health Promotion, and Injury Prevention."

In response to my application, Oakland University invited me to their campus for an interview. Again I wondered how much explaining I would have to do about Loma Linda University. After all it does not have the name recognition of a Harvard, or a Stanford, or a University of Michigan.

During the interview process, I met with the Dean of the School of Health Sciences. As he reviewed my resume he wanted to know if I knew Dr. Joyce Hopp. Again I had to hold onto my seat to avoid falling.

Dr. Hopp was Dean of the School of Allied Health Professions at Loma Linda. Before accepting that position she had been chair of the health education program.

and my instructor in several classes. I learned that this dean of a secular university had rubbed shoulders with her at a number of conferences. The favorable impression she had left in his mind, again spoke highly of Loma Linda University.

Throughout the United States today, scientific interest in the area of wellness and health promotion is growing. Numerous studies are ongoing in the fields of, nutrition, exercise, stress management, and disease prevention. Invariably the data in study after study validates the message God gave to Ellen White in Otsego, Michigan one hundred and fifty years ago in the midst of the American Civil War.

Lifestyle Can Make A Difference — In 1955, forty-two year-old Nathan Pritikin received a death sentence from his physicians. Diagnosed with lymphatic cancer and severe coronary heart disease, he was only given months to live.

His heart specialist told him there was nothing he could do about his blood cholesterol level at 280 mg/dl. (Recommendations are that blood cholesterol levels be below 200). Any exercise, "even walking," was out of the question as he was told it would kill him.

But Mr. Pritikin wasn't ready to die. If the doctors didn't have solutions he would find his own answers. Though a businessman by profession, he began to read the medical literature. What he learned caused him to give up his rich, fatty food diet. He started an exercise program, gradually at first and then more intensely when he found that instead of dropping dead he was actually beginning to feel better.

In time, he began sharing his experience and knowledge with others. In the 1970's he opened the Pritikin Longevity Center in Santa Monica, California. His program of a low-fat, virtually vegetarian diet, along with a regular exercise routine, became legendary throughout the United States. Careful records collected on his clients showed that lifestyle does make a difference, even to the extent of reversing diseases physicians deemed "incurable."

While I was a graduate student at Loma Linda, the Pritikin program was at its apex of success. One of my professors remarked one day that Nathan Pritikin had told him, "I am not doing anything different than what you people have known for 100 years."[13]

The voracity of his dramatic change in lifestyle was vindicated via the autopsy performed after his death at the age of 69. The pathology report stated that the coronary arteries of Pritikin's heart were "as clean as those of a 10-year-old boy."[14]

When men like Nathan Pritikin have nothing but praise for the lifestyle that Adventists have promoted throughout their history, it disturbs me that often we hesitate to proclaim the message too loudly, for fear of rejection by those we are trying to impress. As an example of this, I think of an incident that occurred while I was working at Hong Kong Adventist Hospital. Prior to working there I had spent three years working in tobacco education and stop smoking programs in southern California. During that time, the State of California passed some of the strictest anti-smoking laws in the United States. A movement began that eventually led to the ban on smoking in any public building including bars and nightclubs, establishments usually notorious for their tobacco smoke-filled interiors. As a result, California now has one of the lowest adult smoking rates in the US.

So I was troubled when upon arrival in Hong Kong as the new director of Health Promotion and Wellness, I learned that not only was smoking permitted in the hospital, but it was actually allowed in patients' rooms.

At an administrative council meeting, I made my case for eliminating this health destroying practice. I was told that since smoking was such an ingrained part of the culture, to initiate such a policy would result in a large loss of patients. I reminded the council of the prophet's words written at an earlier time but still applicable today. When the Battle Creek Sanitarium was losing patrons due in part to a decision to no longer serve flesh foods in the dining room she wrote:

"Lately the number of patients at the sanitarium has decreased, owing to an array of circumstances that could not be helped. One reason for the lack of patronage is, I think, the stand that those at the head of the institution have taken against serving flesh meat to the patients. Ever since the opening of the sanitarium, meat has been served in the dining room. We felt that the time had come to take a decided stand against this practice. We knew that it was not pleasing to God for flesh meat to be placed before the patients.

Now no tea, coffee, or flesh meat is served in the institution. We are determined to live out the principles of health reform, to walk in the way of truth and righteousness. We shall not, for fear of losing patronage, be half-and-half reformers. We have taken our position, and by God's help we shall stand by it. ...

Plans must be set in operation that will bring an increase of patronage. But would it be right for us, for the sake of obtaining more patients, to return to the serving of flesh meat? Shall we give the sick that which has made them sick, that which will keep them sick if they continue to use it as food? Shall we not rather take our stand as those who are resolved to carry out the principles of health reform?"[15]

Finally the hospital agreed to set up a committee to assess what other hospitals were doing. The chaplain, who was the head of that committee came back with the report, "Smoking is completely prohibited in all Hong Kong government hospitals."

Now the hospital was willing to gradually wean smoking from the hospital. I pushed for a complete ban on hospital premises. Certain medical facilities in the United States such as the Mayo Clinic were taking that approach. Again I was told it was too radical of a move.

Happily, some twelve years later, patients no longer congregate outside the hospital entrance to puff on their death sticks. Why not? It isn't because of initiatives on behalf of Hong Kong Adventist Hospital. Rather due to an edict of the Hong Kong government that went into effect on January 1, 2007, all hospitals in Hong Kong must impose a smoke-free zone on their entire premises. In fact, except for Singapore, Hong Kong now has the strictest anti-smoking laws in all of Asia. How sad that Adventists were not seen as the catalyst behind such community wide health promotion endeavors.

God told Israel of old, that if they would follow his voice fully, he would make them the head. Yet how often do we follow instead, Israel's penchant for compromise in an attempt to secure worldly approbation?

It sometimes appears that other organizations and institutions are overtaking Adventists when it comes to lifestyle interventions. For 100 years, Adventists were leaders in setting the gold standard when it came to behavior change programs. Now we are losing that distinction to the Nathan Pritikins, the Dean Ornishs, and the Kenneth Coopers. Many in the preventive health arena have chided Adventists for not setting a better example of following our teachings in these matters.

When we as a people have such a beautiful, all inclusive health message, it also disturbs me to see so many Seventh-day Adventists flocking to the newest worldly health fad, whatever it be. Often Adventists seem to be the first to enter some new multilevel marketing scheme based on nutritional supplements, or to jump on some bizarre diet because it has been popularized in the local press. For example, I personally have known Adventists who have gone on a weight loss regimen such as the high-fat, high protein Atkin's Diet which not only has potentially harmful side-effects, but is in direct opposition to the type of diet God gave in Eden.

In many cases our habits of living reflect a craving for the Egyptian way of life — eating the wrong foods, living as couch potatoes, being unduly stressed with so many time pressures, not giving God His rightful priority in our lives. Then when the inevitable results are seen in excess adipose tissue deposited randomly throughout the body,

I believe we add insult to injury by seeking the world's methods of resolution, which in the long term don't work anyway.

One of the most effective methods for helping others to change behaviors, is to use what is known as "modeling." In other words, rather than just lecturing, or quoting a "thus saith the Lord," demonstrate in your own life the desired behavior that you are trying to teach to another. Or to make it even clearer, "Practice what you preach."

Over the years I have been fortunate to come in contact with people who have done just that. And the Lord has richly blessed them for their faithfulness in following His plan. In the next chapter I summarize the lives of three individuals who have been role models for me. By following to the best of their ability the health message that God gave to Seventh-day Adventists, they reached the pinnacle of health and well-being. God indeed *set them on high, above all other peoples of the earth.*

CHAPTER 10

ADVENTISTS WHO MADE A DIFFERENCE

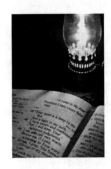

And ye shall be witnesses unto me both in Jeru-salem, and in all Judea, and in Samaria, and unto the uttermost parts of the earth.

Acts 1:8

Introduction — In their first <u>Chicken Soup For the Soul</u> book, Jack Canfield and Mark Hansen tell the following story.

One day a teacher in New York City decided to honor her high school seniors. One by one she called them to the front of the room and told the class what a difference each had made to her. When the last student had been praised, she gave everyone a blue ribbon imprinted with bold gold letters, **"Who I Am Makes A Difference.."**

The students were then given extra ribbons and told to pass them on to others who had made a difference in their lives. One boy went to a junior executive who had helped him with career planning. He explained the school project while pinning a blue ribbon on the man's chest. He then gave him two ribbons and asked him to keep the project going.

Later that day the man went in to see his boss who at times had been difficult to get along with. He explained how he had received a blue ribbon and now he wanted to honor his boss in the same way. "I admire you for your creative genius," he declared while pinning a blue ribbon on him. Before leaving the shocked executive's office, he gave him a second ribbon and asked that he pass it on.

When the executive arrived home that evening he sat down his 14-year-old son. He then told the story of what had happened to him that day. It was obvious he relished the fact that someone had thought enough about him that he would take the time to express his appreciation.

He finished his account by saying, "As I was driving home I began to think of who I could honor. Next to your mother you are the most important person in my life. I know, sometimes I get real busy and don't have much time for you. And sometimes I yell and scream at you because of your grades or your bedroom is a mess. But son, tonight I just wanted to take a moment and tell you how much you mean to me. You're a great kid, I love you, and I want to honor you with this ribbon because **"You Make A Difference."**

The boy began to sob and sob. Large tears coursed down his face while his body convulsed uncontrollably. Looking up through the falling tears he blurted, "I was planning on committing suicide tomorrow, because I didn't think you love me. Now I don't need to."[1]

It is easy to get so caught up in the rapid pace of everyday living, that we neglect to take time to tell people how important they are to us. In this chapter, I want to take the time to highlight a few people who have made a difference in terms of the Adventist health message. More importantly, I want them and their families to know what a difference they have made to me personally.

Before reading further, I urge you to put the book down, find someone who is precious to you, and tell them what a difference they have made in your life. Do it now, before you forget! Do it now, before it is too late! Too often we wait until death to eulogize those we love. Please go and do it now while the loved one can benefit from your words of appreciation. Let that person know that he or she has **made a difference in your life**.

My Adventist Heritage — I was the middle of three siblings. My childhood was spent with an older and a younger sister in Warminster, Pennsylvania, a suburb north of Philadelphia. My grandparents, on my father's side, lived just four miles from us in Willow Grove. I do not remember much about my grandmother because she died from a stroke when I was only six-years-old. I do remember though that she had been very active in Ingathering and in bringing neighborhood children to church.

My grandparents were Episcopalians when they met. They were married in a famous landmark of historical Philadelphia, Old Christ Church. This church dates back to the American Revolution and was the home church of such famous Americans as George Washington, Benjamin Franklin, and Betsy Ross, who designed the first American flag.

Sometime after their wedding, my grandparents took Bible studies and my grandmother was baptized into the Seventh-day Adventist Church. The reason my grandfather did not join the church at this time was probably twofold. First, he was a florist and Saturday was his shop's busiest day of the week. Secondly, he really enjoyed smoking a pipe and cigars. However, many years later, after his retirement, he finally gave up smoking and was baptized when in his seventies.

To my grandmother's credit, all four of her children, my father and three aunts, became baptized members of the Seventh-day Adventist Church. All of them married other Seventh-day Adventists, two of whom became workers for the church, one as an elementary school teacher and the other as a physician.

It was either during my freshman or sophomore year at Columbia Union College, when one day as I was sitting alone in the student lounge, an elderly lady came over and started a conversation. When she found out I was studying theology she became interested in my background.

As the conversation progressed I divulged my last name, "Andress."

"Do you have any relatives in Philadelphia," she next inquired.

I explained that that was my father's childhood home.

She then began to share bits and pieces about some "Andresses" she had known in Philadelphia. The description fit my grandparents perfectly.

Before going on her way she said, "I am sure that it was I who gave Bible studies to your grandmother."

The lady I had met was Ms. Louise Kleuster, author of The Bible Worker, which for many years was the text used to prepare Bible workers in the Seventh-day Adventist denomination. I never saw Mrs. Kleuster again and shortly thereafter she passed away.

You can imagine my surprised elation then, when in August of 2005, I was visiting Elder Carpena in the South Pacific Asian Division headquarters, when upon catching a glimpse of a wall plaque dedicated to Adventist women who made a difference, I saw a photograph of Louise Kleuster.

The Seeds of Mission Service Are Born — During my lifetime, God has brought me in contact with numerous people, who like Mrs. Kleuster, have made a difference in my life. I grew up listening to stories of the early pioneers. The sacrifices that the Whites, Joseph Bates, Uriah Smith. J. N Andrews and others made because of their conviction that Jesus was to soon return, stirred my young soul. In both Sabbath School and elementary school I looked forward to reading the biographies of men like David Livingston, William Carey, Adoniram Judson, Fernando Stahl, and Eric B. Hare; missionary minded men who like Abraham of old, heeded the call of God and went out "not knowing wither they went." Such stories made an indelible impression on my mind and to a large degree are responsible for my decision to spend several years in mission service; some of the best years of my life, I might add.

Many local Seventh-day Adventist churches no longer place an emphasis on missions. Especially in North America, seldom is a weekly mission story recited before the whole Sabbath School. Nor do I hear stories of our pioneers being related today. As a result, many new converts to Adventism have but a dim picture of our rich heritage. This is indeed sad.

In the pages that follow, I briefly summarize the lives of three people who in their personal lives exemplified and followed the health message that God has given to this church. They are living proof that following such teachings can enable one to live well past the three score and ten years that Moses wrote about in the Psalms. I praise God that my pathway through life crossed theirs.

Dr Mervyn Hardinge, M.D., PhD, DrPH— Dean Emeritus of the School of Public Health, Loma Linda University, and former Health and Temperance Secretary of the General Conference of Seventh-day Adventists.

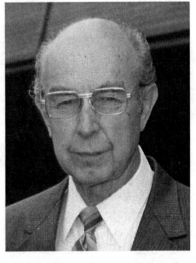

I can think of no individual, who over the last half century, has had more of an influence on the dissemination of the Adventist health message than Mervyn G. Hardinge, M.D. For more than forty years, hundreds of medical students and public health students were privileged to sit in the classroom of this humble, yet erudite, professor. It was in just such a setting that I first met him.

It was the Fall of 1979. I had matriculated in the Master's of Public Health in Health Education program at Loma Linda University. All public health majors were required to take "Philosophy of Health," taught by Dr. Hardinge. It was scheduled as the very first class in the morning. But in a curriculum that included theoretical classes such as "Health Education Planning," and "Public Health Statistics," it was a breath of fresh air. It didn't hurt either that the only course requirements were to attend every class, and not to fall asleep during lectures.

That last stipulation was not too difficult. Dr. Hardinge was not only an excellent teacher, he was also a gifted storyteller. Lectures on exercise, nutrition, water, air, temperance, and mental health were illustrated with practical experiences from his own life. Sitting in his classes I determined that someday, I too would be able to deliver similar scintillating lectures.

I was in the last batch of students to take "Philosophy of Health," from Dr. Hardinge before he retired from teaching in January 1980. Shortly thereafter he was called out of retirement to become the Health and Temperance Director of the General Conference in Silver Springs, Maryland. I probably would not have had any further contact with him, had it not been for an event that happened three years later.

While I was a student at Loma Linda, the School of Health had its own graphics art department. In addition to producing all of the school's advertising materials, the department assisted professors in preparing lecture slides and overheads as this was before the era of personal computers, PowerPoint, and palm size digital video cameras.

I was hired as a departmental assistant, even though my artistic abilities were of such a nature that Dick Croft, the assistant graphic artist, could truthfully state, "Bill, cannot even draw a straight line."

Fortunately there was enough other work so that I could mask my artistic inabilities. My duties included slide and photo copying, reel-to-reel tape editing, producing overheads for instructors, and whatever other menial tasks were required. After completing a correspondence course in photography, I was given additional responsibilities working in the darkroom developing film and enlarging photographs.

One day, Martin Knopper, the graphic arts department director, approached me, "Bill, Dr. Hardinge has received some grant money to update slide-tape programs called the "Hardinge Lifestyle Series." He is looking for a scriptwriter. Would you be interested?"

I had never written an audio-visual script in my life. But by this time I had worked long enough in producing teaching materials that the possibility excited me. I told Mr. Knopper I would submit a script for evaluation.

I'm not sure whether I've retained a copy of that script. It may be buried in a file someplace. More likely it wasn't worth saving. When I think back on it, I conclude that Dr. Hardinge must have been really desperate when he hired me.

For whatever reason, after reading my submission, Dr. Hardinge scheduled an interview with me. I looked forward to it with trepidation. True, I had just completed a double Master's degree program at Loma Linda, but I was going to be sitting face to face with a man who had not one, but three doctorates after his name. First there was the MD from Loma Linda. Next came a Doctor of Public Health from Harvard, followed by a PhD in Pharmacology from Stanford.

Dr. Hardinge was the founder of the School of Health at Loma Linda University, and its first Dean. Nationally he was recognized as a noted researcher, with numerous published articles in peer reviewed journals, particularly in the area of vegetarianism. Oh, and did I mention he was also an ordained minister?

Who was I to even think that I had anything of value to offer? But somewhere, Dr. Hardinge saw some hidden abilities that would be useful in developing materials for health educators. I am grateful for the opportunity he gave me because the next eight years proved to be some of the most meaningful and creative of my professional career.

During the years I worked for him, I found Mervyn G. Hardinge to be one of the humblest, friendliest, most unassuming individuals I have ever known. My work station was located in the same room in which he had his desk and files. I noticed that none of his diplomas were on display as is customary in the offices of professors in university settings. One day while searching for some material for a project we were working on, I found them buried in the bottom drawer of his desk.

That is the type of person he was. Dr. Hardinge frequently rubbed shoulders with the intellectual giants of the world. Yet he made it a practice to never call undue attention to himself, or his myriad noteworthy accomplishments.

As mentioned above, Mervyn (I don't think he minds my using his first name) was a great storyteller. It was a joy to work in an environment where one could be entertained on a regular basis. There were tales of his childhood days in India, canvassing in England, and teaching medicine and public health at Loma Linda. As entertaining as his stories were, he made sure that each was connected to a spiritual object lesson.

One day, I was surprised to hear of "the enemies" in his professional life. When questioned about this he said with a twinkle in his eye, "Oh, yes. I have had my share of enemies, but God has always worked things out for good." He then went on to recount how in his professional obligations he often made "enemies" in committee meetings because of his consistent practice to vote on principle, rather than to be pressured into casting a compromising vote based on what was expedient at the moment.

Shortly before leaving for my mission assignment in Hong Kong, I paid a visit to him. We parted with his words of advice ringing in my ears. "While in Hong Kong you will be asked to sit on various committees. There will be times in which you will be under tremendous pressure to vote along with the crowd. If there is some reason why in good conscience you cannot agree with the majority, then don't vote with them just for convenience sake. Always cast your vote according to principle. It may cost you in the near term, but in the end God will work it out for your good."

In the intervening years, I have sat on many committees. I have never been able to vote on an issue without those words resounding again and again in the inner recesses of my brain. In hindsight I can see that it was sound, solid advice.

At the time I started working for Dr. Hardinge, the role of Ellen White as a prophet, was being called into question within the church. It was a time when Dr. Desmond Ford, a theology professor at Pacific Union College was questioning Adventist teachings on the sanctuary. Then a former Adventist pastor, Walter Rhea, published a book disparaging the Gift of Prophecy called, "The White Lie."

As Health and Temperance Secretary for the General Conference, Dr. Hardinge was able to feel the full impact of those assaults. He had a great burden to answer some of the charges being made and elected to do so through the medium of an audio-visual production. The result was *"By Voice and Pen,"* a 12-minute slide-tape program documenting how God led in the life of Ellen White and her contributions to a Seventh-day Adventist understanding of healthful living.

The church also felt a need to revise and update its "Five-Day Plan to Quit Smoking." The "Five-Day Plan to Quit Smoking," usually shortened to "The Five-Day Plan," was started in 1960 by two men, Dr. J. Wayne MacFarland, a medical doctor who happened to be my Sabbath-School teacher in my early teens, and Elmer Folkenberg, a pastor. It is significant to note that not only was this the first group therapy approach to helping people quit smoking, but the inaugural program was conducted four years before the US government came out with the first Surgeon General's Report on Smoking and Health documenting the dangers associated with tobacco smoke.

Prior to its publication, smoking rates among the American adult male population exceeded 40%. In the 1950's and 1960's, many physicians themselves were smokers. Smoking advertisements on both TV and radio were frequent. It was easy for young kids to pick up the catchy jingles. The Marlboro cowboy became the most successful advertising campaign in history, and to this day I can remember the slogan connected with its advertisements.

Within a period of years, "The 5-Day Plan" had become so successful that it was endorsed around the world by such organizations as the World Health Organization and the American Heart Association. At one time, all subsequent group therapy programs that utilized behavior modification techniques, based their programs on fundamentals of "The 5-Day Plan."

But 20 years after its inception, the church realized a need for revision and refinement. Since the "Five-Day Plan" was conceived, the scientific studies documenting the dangers of smoking had proliferated Furthermore, it was recognized that breaking addictions was a complicated process and that a multifaceted approach was needed to reach a varied population. Thus in the mid-1980's the original "5-Day Plan," was updated with the new "Breathe Free" program. Dr. Hardinge was commissioned to produce 10 audio-visual programs to supplement the new material.

Dr. Hardinge's operation within the Department of Health Education became known as Healthstyle Productions. Its mission was to produce educational materials that could be used by laymen and health professionals alike. In addition to the stop smoking programs, the "Hardinge Lifestyle Series" label included programs on exercise, nutrition, sleep, natural remedies, and other components of the Adventist lifestyle. In total, some twenty-five programs were produced, ranging in length from 12–20 minutes.

A great burden of Dr. Hardinge's was to disseminate the Adventist health message worldwide. He recognized the importance of giving a global appeal to the programs. In this aspect he was ahead of the times in building ethnic diversity into the script and the accompanying illustrative slides. Sometimes, for those of us responsible for the actual production, this could be rather frustrating. Yet Dr. Hardinge remained undeterred in designing content that would appeal to a global church.

On one occasion he returned from Panama where he had just conducted an evangelistic series with then General Conference President, Neal Wilson. While there he had pilot tested several new programs we were readying for production. Upon his return he was adamant that we reshoot a picture depicting various fruit options, "You need to include bananas and coconuts. People in the developing world cannot afford the fruits depicted in this slide."

We had no choice but to take the time to set up the shot again, and this time include the appropriate tropical fruits. "You need to include bananas and coconuts," became our catch phrase when evaluating future programs for their ethnic diversity content. We knew that if a program lacked appeal to varied ethnic groups, Dr. Hardinge would make us edit and re-edit until it achieved such a focus.

A man whom I have come to regard as one of my dearest and closest friends, Art Mallon, was hired to market the programs. Whereas we had been use to selling one or two programs at a time, Art amazed us by ringing up sets of 10-12 programs in one sale. Through the utilization of his marketing skills, the "Hardinge Lifestyle Series" was distributed worldwide.

When I arrived in Hong Kong in 1993, most of the Hardinge Lifestyle Programs had preceded me to the Wellness/Health Promotion office. Seven years later I found myself teaching at the Adventist International Institute of Advanced Studies in the Philippines. Once again, this time in the audio-visual section of the library, I saw a set of the Hardinge Lifestyle Programs. Many of these programs have since been translated into Spanish, German, and other languages. While I was in Hong Kong, a number of them were translated into Cantonese.

The last major undertaking of Healthstyle Productions before it closed in 1990, was the video taping of Dr. Hardinge's 10-part trademark lecture series, "*Philosophy of Health*" Through these tapes, Dr. Hardinge continues to reach thousands of professionals and laymen alike with the passion of his life, "restoring in man the image of God, physically, mentally, and spiritually."

Somehow it seems fitting that my professional connection with this crusader of healthful living ended where it began — listening to him share the great principles of health and wellness. Thank you Dr. Hardinge for your commitment to the Adventist heritage of health, and for making a difference in my life.*

Mrs. Hulda Crooks — Oldest person to climb Mt. Whitney, the highest mountain in the continental United States, and oldest woman and American to climb Mt. Fuji, Japan's highest peak. Both feats were accomplished at the age of 91.

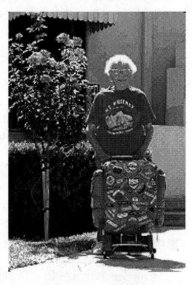

"How would you like an assistant to help you in your research," asked Mr. Knopper.

The year was 1982. We had almost finished producing the first program in the Hardinge Lifestyle Series. Dr. Hardinge had provided me with some rough drafts for the next several programs on nutrition and they needed to be documented. I was glad for the offer to have someone help me with the research.

A couple of days later I was introduced to my "research assistant," a white haired grandmotherly type in her eighties.

---

* To learn more about this remarkable God-fearing man I suggest readers obtain his autobiography: Hardinge, Mervyn G. *My Unexpected Life.* TEACH Services Inc., Brushton, New York, 2005.

"Come on, give me a break," I thought to myself. "This project requires graduate research. Don't give me someone who may know how to type, but is probably at best in the early stages of Alzheimer's."

Fortunately, I kept my thoughts to myself. Yet, I decided to

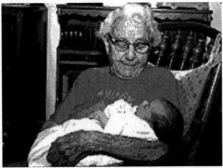

One of my favorite photos. Ninety-year-old Hulda Crooks cradles my three-week-old daughter.

validate my impressions by giving her an assignment. "Mrs. Crooks," I said mustering as much politeness in my voice as possible, "Dr. Hardinge wants to make several programs on protein. I need information on the following men: Justus von Liebig, Karl Voit, Hindhede, Russell Chittenden, and Henry Sherman."

To be honest, I knew virtually nothing about those individuals. Oh, I had been exposed to the names in classes like Philosophy of Health and Public Health Nutrition, but frankly all I remembered was that they had made some sort of contribution in the field of nutrition. I was sure that Mrs. Crooks would come back empty-handed on this request.

"When do you need the data," she asked.

Feeling that I better give her plenty of time I answered, "If you can have the information within a week, that should be fine."

The next morning when I came into my office, sitting on my desk was a folder containing detailed descriptions of each of those men. All the information I needed was there, neatly arranged in chronological order.

A short time later, I needed Mrs. Crooks help again. This time she replied, "I don't think I can find this material in Dr. Hardinge's files. I will need to go to the library. It will probably take me a little longer to find what you need."

And it did; about two or three days longer. But once again she was able to retrieve the precise data and references that I needed.

How completely wrong, ill-informed pre-conceived judgments can be!

I decided I better find out a bit about this woman who had shattered my stereotyping of the elderly. I discovered that for 30 years, Hulda Crooks had been Dr. Hardinge's personal secretary. No one knew the contents of the six, 4-drawer file cabinets in his office as well as she did.

I also learned that this lady had developed quite a bit of notoriety in southern California for her exploits on the mountains in the area. Near Palm Springs, 50 miles east of Loma Linda, were the highest of the southern California mountains, Mt. San Jacinto and Mt. San Gorgonio. Both towered over 10,500 feet (3,180 meters). She had trekked to their summits on several occasions.

But Mrs. Crooks was best known for her annual climb up 14,497 foot (4,392 meters) Mt. Whitney. Located in the southern Sierra Nevada range which runs down the back of California, it is the tallest mountain in the United States, outside of Alaska.

Hulda first climbed it when she was 66-years-old. She had climbed it every year since except one year when bad weather had turned her back before reaching the summit. She always let her listeners know that she had made up for that failure by climbing it twice one summer. Other exploits included hiking to the bottom of the Grand Canyon at age 75 and backpacking the entire 212 mile (340 kilometer) John Muir Trail over the course of five summers. The high altitude trail meanders along the granite peaks and wildflower filled alpine valleys of the Sierra Nevada from Yosemite to Sequoia National Park. Mt. Whitney lies at the southern terminus of that trail. I also learned she held the 10K running record for women over the age of 80.

Obviously this woman was as physically fit as she was mentally alert. So I quickly grabbed the opportunity to be part of the team that would accompany her on her 21st. climb of Mt. Whitney.

Even though reaching Mt. Whitney's peak involved a 22-mile roundtrip high altitude climb, half of it with a full backpack, I figured that if an 87-year-old lady could do it, then it couldn't be all that difficult.

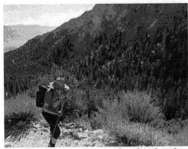

Hulda Crooks leisurely climbs the first leg of the Mt. Whitney Trail.

Once again, bad judgment on my part. My muscles quickly rebelled at carrying the 45-pound pack. Crossing the first mountain stream, I lost both my balance and my ego, on the slippery rocks and fell in. In all her jaunts up Whitney, Hulda never fell; not even once.

The next day it rained. The higher we climbed the worse the rain got. By the time I pitched my tent at Trail Camp (12,000 feet) I was soaking wet. I was tired. And I was cold. To make matters worse, the tent leaked, from both the top and the bottom. I could not envision spending another night on that horrible mountain under those miserable conditions.

When Dick, my tent mate, and several others disclosed their plans for evacuation, I quickly struck the tent so I could pack out with them. Several hours later we made it back to our cars parked at the Whitney Portal. The comforts of home were only a four and a half hour drive away. Hulda could

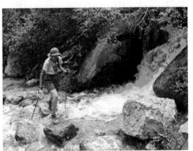

My sister, Nancy fords Lone Pine Creek. This was the stream I fell into on my first climb up Whitney.

have her "fun excursions" on Whitney. I had had enough of the mountain and swore that I would never go near it again.

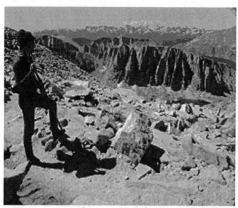

A view near the crest of the Mt. Whitney Trail.

Six weeks later, my resolve was broken. This time I reached the granite carved inscription that designates it as the highest mountain in California. Once there I viewed the magnificent vistas extending to the horizon in every direction, and understood why Hulda had kept coming back year after year. As she was fond of saying, "Once you have been to the mountaintop, the valleys don't look so difficult."

That was another characteristic of Hulda; her upbeat attitude. Hers had not been an easy life. When at the age of 18, she decided to become a Seventh-day Adventist, her father told her to leave home and never come back again. All she had were a few dresses, less than five dollars, and a fifth grade education.

In her early adulthood she was often sickly. Her husband, Sam, suggested she do gardening and go hiking in an attempt to regain her health. As she became stronger, she began to conquer both physical and personal mountains.

Then the only man whom she had ever fallen in love with, suddenly passed away from heart failure. While still adjusting to widowhood, her only son tragically died from a drug overdose. No, Hulda endured more than her fair share of hardship. Yet she was never known to wear a frown or harbor discontent or discouragement.

Her life was governed by a deep abiding trust in God. Her most cherished possession was the well-worn Bible which her husband, Sam, had given to her as an engagement present. She knew the God of that Book and began each day by spending time with Him. The faith thus developed through life's experiences and her daily devotions exuded from her smile and words of encouragement.

By the time I started climbing with her, Hulda Crooks had become a household name to climbers across America. Whenever she was on the Whitney Trail, the word would quickly spread up and down the mountain, "Hulda is here. Hulda is here."

While in camp she was never too busy to chat with other hikers and to give them words of hope and encouragement. She had a small tract printed up detailing her philosophy of health. These she carried in her backpack and passed out by the thou-

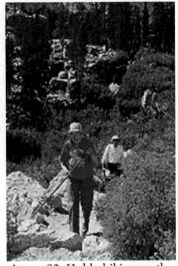

At age 92, Hulda hiking on the Mt. Whitney trail to Outpost Camp for the last time.

sands. Her "high altitude evangelism" resulted in several baptisms over the years. I still meet people today who credit their current state of health and spirituality to an encounter they had with Hulda Crooks.

In 1987, Dentsu, Japan's largest advertising firm, heard about Hulda's exploits. They invited her to join them in their 60th annual trek up Mt. Fuji, Japan's highest mountain. I believe the highlight of my life was accompanying her on that trip.

On Friday morning, July 24, 1987, she huddled in the frigid mountain air,

Hulda prepares to pass through one of the Shinto gates that mark the Mt. Fuji Trail.

as the first rays of sunlight emerged from a deep red orb rising above the clouds over the Pacific Ocean. Four hundred Dentsu employees raised their hands in salute as they shouted *"Banzai, Banzai* — To your health."* At the age of 91, Hulda had become the oldest woman and the oldest American to climb their sacred mountain and they rejoiced with her in her success.

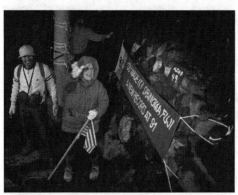

Reaching the summit of Mt. Fuji at 3:45 a.m., July 24, 1987.

Later that evening, her story was broadcast around the world, when on ABC Nightly News, Peter Jennings featured her as "The Person of the Week." And just six weeks later she broke her own record as the oldest person to climb Mt. Whitney. As of this writing, both of these records still stand.

Her last visit to the Whitney Wilderness area was in 1991. Jerry Lewis, a longtime friend of hers in the United States Congress had arranged for her to be flown to Trail Camp in a Chinook military helicopter. This was the very place I had turned back on my first trek up the mountain.

Upon arrival, in the shadow of Mt. Whitney's granite profile, Congressman Lewis read the following congressional proclamation. "The second peak south of Mt. Whitney, the highest peak of Pinnacle Ridge, shall be known and designated as Crooks Peak."

Official letters including one from President George Bush Sr. were then read, "You have not only highlighted the importance of physical fitness for all Americans, but also served as a role model for senior citizens everywhere."

She not only was a role model in terms of living, but I believe she was a role model in death as well. Many young people and adults approaching middle age are afraid of the aging process. They envision a slow deterioration in which their bodies are filled with aches and pains and they are no longer capable of doing the things they once enjoyed. To a large degree Mrs. Crooks challenged that stereotype.

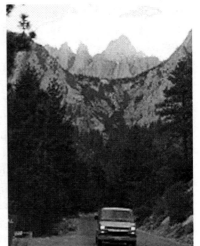

Mt. Whitney as seen from the road leading to Whitney Portal. Crooks' Peak is the spire to the far left

Before going to Japan, I assisted in giving her a stress test on the treadmill. The results showed that she had a physical fitness level typical of someone 25 years younger.

I last visited Hulda about three months before her death. While no longer climbing mountains she was still ambulatory and quite independent. She told me, "I don't have any pain but I tire easily. I am ready to go. I am ready to go to sleep and wait for the second coming with my beloved Sam."

My promise to her was that someday I would break her Whitney record. However, as with each passing birthday I feel myself yielding to the aging process, I understand better what an incredible feat it was to be able to climb so high at her age. As a matter of fact, in July of 2006, I climbed with my sister and brother-in-law. They had never been on the mountain before. In fact, other than Mt. Fuji on their honeymoon, they had never climbed anything taller than the 6,000 foot highpoints found in the Appalachian Mountains. My sister succeeded in summiting, but due to a foot injury I sustained, I turned around about a mile short of the top. At age 54, I had gained a new appreciation of what Hulda had really done by successfully climbing the mountain year after year in her seventies and eighties.

Hulda quietly passed away on November 23, 1997 after a very brief illness. Buried in Loma Linda, next to her dear Sam, she awaits the moment when Christ will call both of them forth to be reunited for eternity.

On December 7, 1997, Loma Linda University Church, which seats over 2000, was filled to capacity with those who had in one way or another been touched by Hulda's life. They had come to pay their final tribute to this remarkable woman. Illustrative of how far reaching that influence had been was Mr. Tsuneo Kuromizu, Dentsu's Public Relations officer, who flew all the way from Japan to pay the respects of his company and his country.

The following summer, Mr. Kuromizu invited me to again join Dentsu's annual trek up Fujisan. In the Sengen Shinto shrine, atop the mountain, I was given the honor of presenting a plaque to the head priest, commemorating Hulda's record of eleven years earlier. Beneath a photo of Hulda setting that record, the following testimony is engraved in both English and Japanese.

"On July 24, 1987, at 3:45 am, Mrs. Hulda Crooks, Ambassador of Healthful Living, from Loma Linda, California, USA, became the oldest woman and the oldest American to successfully climb Japan's highest and most sacred mountain, Fuji.

This plaque accepted by the Sengen Shrine atop Mt. Fuji on the first anniversary of the historic climb following her ascension stands as a memorial to the indefatigable human spirit and is dedicated to all who follow in her footsteps in reaching the summit."

Signed — Dentsu Inc, July 24, 1998.

The theology may be flawed but the reverence and esteem the people of Japan bestowed on this humble woman is clear. What a tribute to the witness of an unassuming woman who never dreamed that obedience to

God's health principles would bring such world renown. What a testimony to our God, that in this land of non-Christians, a plaque honoring a Seventh-day Adventist should reside in a Shinto shrine atop Japan's most sacred mountain.

Such was the international influence of one solitary woman. Thank you Hulda for being a vibrant testimony to healthful living and for making a difference in my life too.†

Harry Miller, M.D. — Personal physician to military leaders, emperors, and presidents. Also the founder of some 20 hospitals throughout Asia.

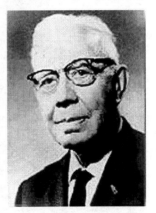

Sometimes individuals have an indirect influence on our lives. Such was the influence of Harry Willis Miller on mine.

For the six years I lived in Hong Kong, I resided in the La Rue Villa. This was a twelve story building whose 36 apartments had been designed to house expatriate workers at Hong Kong Adventist Hospital. The complex was directly across the driveway from the hospital entrance. With land at a premium, buildings tend to be crowded together in Hong Kong. They also reach upward rather than outward. As we were preparing to leave Hong Kong, construction had begun on a building two doors away from the hospital. It has since been completed and at over 70 stories high is the tallest residential building in the world.

---

† To learn more about this remarkable God-fearing woman I suggest readers obtain her brief biography: Andress, William C. and Goede, Winnie. *Grandma Whitney: Queen of the Mountain.* TEACH Services, Inc. Brushton, New York, 1996.

The La Rue Villa was named after Abraham La Rue, the first Seventh-day Adventist missionary to Asia. Abraham was not a pastor nor did he have any formal theological training. By occupation he was a shepherd and woodcutter. In middle age he joined the Seventh-day Adventist Church and immediately began to share the three angels' messages with all he came in contact with.

Having a special burden for the Chinese living in mainland China, he requested that the General Conference send him there as a missionary. They flatly refused his request telling him that since he was in his mid-sixties, he was too old.

But La Rue was persistent. Finally in more of an attempt to get him off their backs than in appreciation

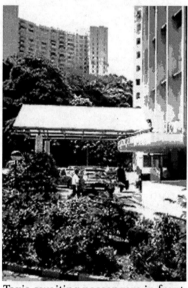

for his missionary zeal, the brethren agreed that he could go as a missionary, but he would have to choose some island for his witnessing. China was simply too big and too challenging for an aged worker. Obviously they felt safe in this proposal assuming that La Rue would opt for some relatively easy field such as Hawaii.

La Rue went home and pulled out an atlas. "Hmm," he surmised. "Hong Kong was an island. That's where he would ask to be sent."

Taxis awaiting passengers in front of Hong Kong Adventist Hospital.

And so with great reluctance, Abraham La Rue received the blessing of church leadership to sail on a steamship for the island of Hong Kong, just off the southeast China mainland. In Hong Kong, La Rue began visiting the ships that came into port. To anyone interested he would pass out gospel literature. Thus his missionary influence extended beyond the one small island he was assigned to. In time, Abraham La Rue personally introduced Adventism to a number of Asian countries including Malaysia, Sri Lanka, and the Philippines.

We were assigned to a flat on the 10th floor of the La Rue Villa complex. Never have I had a job where my home was so conveniently located to work. In the morning I would step onto the elevator which was just a few steps from my doorway. Upon reaching ground level I would walk across the driveway, enter the hospital, and take another elevator up to my fifth floor office. Halfway through our term, the Health Promotion and Wellness Department was moved to the fourth floor of the La Rue Villa making it less than a one minute commute from office to home.

Three men were largely responsible for seeing that Hong Kong Adventist Hospital became a reality. They were Ezra Longway, Robert Milne and Harry Miller. Elder Longway and Dr. Miller had passed away long before our arrival, but Pastor Robert Milne was still alive, though in failing health. At the time I was not particularly interested in the detailed history of Adventist institutions. It is a regret I carry to this day, as I realize I missed out on an opportunity to gain some firsthand insight from this missionary who had worked side by side with Dr. Miller.

Dr. Miller gave sixty years of his life to mission service in the Orient. As a lad he grew up on an Ohioan farm. After graduating from Mt. Vernon Academy he followed the advice of Dr. Daniel H. Kress and enrolled at the American Medical Missionary College in Battle Creek, Michigan. One of his professors was none other than John Harvey Kellogg. Reflecting on those classes at Battle Creek he stated, "Perhaps the greatest thing I learned from Dr. John Harvey Kellogg and Dr. David Paulson was the importance of preventive medicine. They taught that if disease can be prevented then it doesn't need to be cured."

As Dr. Miller was nearing the end of his medical internship, the Foreign Mission Board of Seventh-day Adventists asked him, along with his wife Maude who also was a physician, to serve as missionaries in China. When Dr. Kellogg got wind of their plans, he determined to dissuade them from pursuing a course that he deemed to be folly. Kellogg just didn't understand why such an astute young man with a promising career ahead of him in one of America's prestigious medical schools, would relinquish it all on a hardship tour in a mysterious faraway land.

Like Moses who chose to give up the pleasures of Egypt to suffer affliction with the people of God, Harvey and Maude went forth believing that "He who began a good work in them, was able to finish it." Before Dr. Miller's life came to an end at the age of ninety-seven, he would minister to kings, princes, generals, and presidents as well as to the poor and social outcasts of more than fifty countries.

Maude was not as fortunate. After only seventeen months in China she was stricken with a mysterious intestinal illness. A cure eluded her and she died when only 25-years-old. Harry was grief stricken. Now more alone than ever in a strange land, he tried to ease the loss by burying himself in his work. But work alone could not fill the empty void in his heart. On his first furlough back to the United States he met a girl from Maine, Marie. After a short courtship, they married.

Marie was delighted to return to China with her new husband. After a few years it was Harry's turn to be stricken with the debilitating disease that had killed his first wife. The bouts of diarrhea, intestinal inflammation, liver atrophy, and ulceration of the oral cavity slowly but surely weakened the doctor.

A decision to return to his childhood farm in Ohio saved Harry's life. The undiagnosed illness is known today as sprue. It is caused by a deficiency of B vitamins, which were largely lacking in the typical Chinese diet based largely on white rice. Back on the farm he was able to eat an abundance of fruits, whole grains, and vegetables; just the prescription needed for recovery.

While in the United States, Dr. Miller was petitioned by the board of Washington Sanitarium and Hospital to become its medical superintendent. The hospital located on the edge of the nation's capital, was teetering on the brink of bankruptcy so it was with great reluctance that Miller accepted the position. Through hard work and astute judgment, not only did he save the institution, but he turned it into a facility that attracted congressmen, senators, and Supreme Court justices.

I am grateful for his success in that endeavor, for some 30 years later, in the spring of 1952, it was in the maternity ward that I made my entrance into this world. Later I completed my undergraduate studies on the campus of Columbia Union College, located directly across from the hospital grounds. I could look out the front of the men's dorm, across the campus, and see the building where I was born.

While in Washington D.C., Miller served as a consulting physician to two presidents, William Howard Taft, and Woodrow Wilson. It was also during this time that Miller started his career in delicate thyroid surgery.

He became so proficient in this specialization that he gained worldwide acclaim as one of the most skilled thyroid doctors. In performing over 6,000 thyroidectomies, he experienced only a 1% fatality rate, a record virtually unheard of in an age when as many as one out of two thyroid surgery patients could be expected to die.

Despite his success in America, the land of China kept beckoning for his return. Returning in 1925, Dr. Miller spent the bulk of the next 50 years opening hospitals, ministering to the poor, and treating some of Asia's elite.

A regular visitor to the Shanghai Sanitarium was Madame Chiang Kai-shek, wife of the ruler of the Nationalist Party. Raymond Moore in the Preface to his biography of Miller called, <u>China Doctor</u>, states that "he treated nearly every important ruler of China from the founding of the Republic."

But Miller's work in Asia was not limited to China. He frequently traveled to the Philippines to operate there.

Many of his fees were given to help establish the Manila Sanitarium. To expand his realm of influence, Miller sat for, and passed the medical exam with the third highest mark. In the area of surgery he scored 100%, the first person in the history of the Philippine Medical Boards to obtain a perfect score in any subject.

Twenty years later he passed the British medical exam in Canada. This license allowed him to practice medicine in any of the British colonies. In Japan he helped establish Tokyo Adventist Hospital. Asked to stay by and help on a temporary basis, he sat for the Japanese medical exams.

He was able to pass the written part without much difficulty, but was extremely nervous about the oral part, even though it was to be given in English. His nervousness was heightened upon learning that the material he would be tested on pertained to biochemistry. This was one of the doctor's weakest areas and he was fearful that his ignorance here would cause him to fail the test.

When it came his turn, inexplicably the examiner asked him to explain the action of thyroxine, a hormone secreted by the thyroid gland. No one knew the thyroid better than Dr. Miller. The thoroughness and completeness of his answer enabled the Japanese professor to announce that on that exam the "oldest passed best of all."

Following in the footsteps of Dr. Kellogg, his former professor at the American College of Medical Evangelists, Harry Miller developed a keen interest in nutrition. In China, thousands of babies were dying annually due to allergies and nutritional deficiencies. For example, most Asians lack lactase, an enzyme necessary to break down lactose, the sugar in milk. Without the enzyme, the consumption of milk and other dairy products leads to the production of gas, bloating, and diarrhea. For those Chinese mothers who couldn't produce enough breast milk, oftentimes the only alternative was to watch their babies die.

Dr. Miller's concern for these unnecessary deaths led him to develop formulas for producing milk from the soybean. In America, these formulas were marketed under the names of Soyagen and Soyalac. The nutritional composition of these products enabled soy milk to be used as a highly suitable substitute for animal milks and thereby bypass the problems associated with lactase deficiencies.

Today, soy milk industries proliferate in Asia. One of the largest companies is Vitasoy. It is my understanding that the founder of the company obtained his knowledge from Dr. Miller, himself.

Dr. Harry Miller was ninety-one when the Stubbs Road Hong Kong Adventist Hospital opened its doors in May 1971. This was the second hospital he started in Hong Kong. Several years earlier, he and Ezra Longway raised the money to start Tsuen Wan Adventist Hospital on the border between Hong Kong and the New Territories, a kind of buffer zone between Hong Kong and the China mainland. Its targeted population was mainly the thousands of Chinese refugees who were pouring into Hong Kong daily to escape the communist regime of Mao Tse Tung.

One day, Mr. Chan Shun, a wealthy Hong Kong shirt manufacturer, pulled Miller aside and reasoned with him that since most of the money for the hospitals that Dr. Miller started had come from wealthy donors, shouldn't there be a hospital dedicated to this

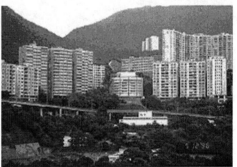

Surrounded by high rises on the road to Victoria Peak, the circular Hong Kong Adventist Hospital has a unique design and is situated in a prominent location.

class of people as well? The indefatigable Harry Miller agreed.

With costs prohibitive and land at a premium, it was voted that the Stubbs Road Mission property would be turned into a hospital. Chan Shun gave a $1,000,000 gift to start the building project. And once again Dr. Miller could take credit for being the catalyst behind the opening of another Adventist medical facility to serve the people of the Orient, in particular, the Chinese.

Two decades later, I would spend some of my most memorable days working as the Director of Health Promotion and Wellness in that facility. The round design of the hospital is unique in its construction and beckons to thousands of Hong Kongers who can easily gaze upon it from across Happy Valley. Situated halfway up the main road to Victoria Peak, the premier tourist spot in Hong Kong, it is a witness to thousands from around the world, everyday.

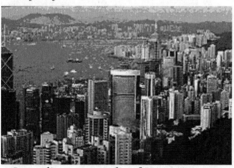
Sprawling metropolis of Hong Kong as seen from Victoria Peak

Its reputation is such that when in the 1990's President Bill Clinton passed through Hong Kong, the United States embassy designated Hong Kong Adventist Hospital as the premier emergency site, in case the president needed medical assistance during his visit. And when the former President of the Philippines, Joseph Estrada, needed surgery while under house arrest, the Philippine government repeatedly refused his requests to have the surgery done in America for fear he would seek asylum there. Instead permission was granted for American doctors to come to Hong Kong and perform the operation at Hong Kong Adventist Hospital.

Hong Kong and its people will always hold a special place in my heart. It has a vibrancy and a pulse that can be experienced in very few other places on the planet.

Thank you Dr. Miller for your vision in establishing Hong Kong Adventist Hospital. Because of your dedication to God and a desire to prevent illness, unbeknownst to you, you made a difference in my life.‡

---

‡　To learn more about this remarkable physician I suggest readers obtain his biography: Moore, Raymond S.: *China Doctor: The Life Story of Harry Willis Miller.* Pacific Press Publishing Association, Boise, Idaho, 1969. (Unfortunately the book is out of print. Used copies are often available through such internet resources as E-bay.)

Chapter 11

"ALL WE GET TO EAT IS MANNA!"

Now all these things happened to them as examples, and they are written for our admonition, upon whom the ends of the ages have come.

I Corinthians 10:11

March 5, 1984 — Loma Linda, California — "You Seventh-day Adventists are the role model for rest of the world," thus declared Dr. William Foege, M.D.[1]

Dr. William Herbert Foege was no ordinary man. He held many prominent positions in his lifetime, perhaps most noteworthy that of director of the Center for Disease Control in Atlanta, Georgia under both Presidents Jimmy Carter and Ronald Reagan. Now while addressing an audience of medical professionals at the annual School of Public Health alumni meetings he was giving recognition to the worldwide influence of Seventh-day Adventist health work.

Such a declaration, by a man of his distinction, places a tremendous responsibility upon Seventh-day Adventists to live up to that reputation. This book began by focusing on ancient Israel, a people whom God had destined to be the epitome of health and wellness: spiritually, mentally, and physically. Yet because of rebellion and obstinate persistence in making wrong choices, they never became that designated role model. Notice:

"When God led the children of Israel out of Egypt, it was His purpose to establish them in the land of Canaan a pure, happy, healthy people....

160

Had they been willing to deny appetite in obedience to His restrictions, feebleness and disease would have been unknown among them. Their descendants would have possessed physical and mental strength. They would have had clear judgment. But they were unwilling to submit to God's requirements, and they failed to reach the standard He had set for them, and to receive the blessings that might have been theirs."[2]

In I Corinthians 10, the apostle Paul declares that the experiences of the Israelites in their journey from Egypt to Canaan were recorded for the benefit of those living in the final days of earth's history. *"Now all these things happened to them as examples, and they are written for our admonition, upon whom the ends of the ages have come"* I Corinthians 10:11. Thus it behooves us to take another look at that record for if we do not learn the lessons of the past we are likely to repeat its mistakes. Could it be that we too are missing out on God's blessings because of a failure to adhere to the physiological laws of our own well-being?

The story of Israel's deliverance from Egyptian bondage is recorded in the first 15 chapters of the book of Exodus with the climax taking place in chapter 14. Hemmed in by physical barriers in front of them and to either side; and with Pharaoh's elite cadre of militia in hot pursuit, Israel faced impending slaughter. There was no way out! That is, until God performed a miracle.

A Song of Victory — Chapter 14 closes with the parting of the Red Sea whereupon the Israelites passed through on dry ground while their pursuers met a watery grave when the walls of water came cascading down upon them. Immediately following, they sang a song of victory as recorded in Exodus 15. It is the song of Moses and the redeemed. *"Then Moses and the children of Israel sang this song to the Lord..."*

It is a song of triumph over Israel's enemies. *"I will sing to the Lord, For He has triumphed gloriously! The*

*horse and its rider He has thrown into the sea. The Lord is
my strength and song, and He has become my salvation."*

It is a song that enticed Miriam and all the Israelite
women to pick up timbrels and lead the encampment in
celebratory dance. *"Then Miriam the prophetess, the sister
of Aaron, took the timbrel in her hand; and all the women
went out after her with timbrels and with dances."*

It is a song that reverberated across the desert sands
as hundreds of thousands of voices proclaimed the glorious triumph of Lord God Almighty. It is a song that cast
fear into Israel's enemies. *"The people will hear and be
afraid; Sorrow shall take hold of the inhabitants of Philis-
tia. Then the chiefs of Edom will be dismayed; the mighty
men of Moab, Trembling will take hold of them; All the
inhabitants of Canaan will melt away. Fear and dread will
fall on them."*

And it is a song that within days, Israel entirely forgot.

Yes, in just three days, Israel forgot the miracle of her
deliverance from bondage. How similar to my experience, and perhaps yours. God works mightily in my behalf. Perhaps in answer to prayer He even performs a
miracle. Yet what happens but a few days later when I'm
confronted with the next obstacle? Too often my trust in
divine outcomes has a tendency to waver when brought
into strait circumstances.

The journey to Canaan had just begun and already
the water jugs were empty. The Israelites may have spent
the last couple of hundred years as slaves in Egypt, but
they knew that one does not attempt to cross a vast desert
without water. To further dampen their faith and trust,
when they did find an oasis at Marah, the water was un-
drinkable.

But man's extremities are God's opportunities. There
at Marah, He turned their mourning into mirth by performing a miracle that transformed the bitter into something better.

In the verse immediately following this experience,
we read, *"If you diligently heed the voice of the Lord your*

God, and do what is right in His sight, give ear to His commandments, and keep all His statutes, I will put none of the diseases on you which I have brought on the Egyptians. For I am the Lord who heals you." Exodus 15:26

This is the first recorded communication that took place between God and Israel after the crossing of the Red Sea. Notice that it was a message pertaining to their physical health.

Now fast forward in your mind to May 21, 1863. You'll recall that that was the day the Seventh-day Adventist Church was formally organized with about 3,500 members. Two weeks later, on Friday evening, June 5, during sundown worship in the little town of Otsego, Michigan, Ellen White received the comprehensive health vision. In it were laid out ten foundational principles that formed the basis for the Seventh-day Adventist Church's teachings on health.

To make sure you get the connection, I repeat. The first message given to Israel after deliverance from Egypt was a message regarding the care of their physical bodies. In 1863, God's remnant church was formally organized. The first vision God gave to the prophet after this organization was a message regarding physical health.

And I would suggest that in the final days of this earth's history, healthful living will again fulfill a prominent place in God's plan. God is going to have a people who can physically withstand the stresses and strains of modern-day living. He will have a people who have the stamina to proclaim the gospel with power, and conviction, and zeal. God needs messengers today who are not physically exhausted and sickly. He needs men and women who are not diseased and dying prematurely because of their wrong habits of living.

In Deuteronomy 4:40 and again in Deuteronomy 5:33 the Bible clearly states that it is possible to extend one's life by obeying God's laws. *"You shall therefore keep His statutes and His commandments, which I command you today, that it may go well with you and with your chil-*

*dren after you, **that you may prolong your days in the land....***"

*"You shall walk in all the ways which the Lord your God has commanded you, that you may live, and **that it may be well with you, and that you may prolong your days*** in the land which you shall possess."*

On the other hand, Ecclesiastes 8:13 indicates that disobedience leads to premature death. *But **it shall not be well with the wicked, nor will he prolong his days**... because he does not fear before God.*

If these texts are not clear enough consider these additional inspired words, *"It is just as much a sin against God to disobey the laws of our being as it is to break one of the ten commandments."*[3]

Returning to the story of the Exodus. In Exodus 15:26 God gave a wondrous promise to the Israelites. But immediately after that, they started to engage in what would become their favorite pastime: catastrophizing and complaining. It made no difference that just days before, God had wrought deliverance from their severe Egyptian taskmasters. Memories of the parting of the Red Sea seem to have been forgotten. The same could be said of the miracle wrought at Marah. One would imagine that if God could provide water for them in the desert then he certainly had the means for feeding them. But no! In the predicament of the present, Israel forgot the Provider of the past.

"Then the whole congregation of the children of Israel complained against Moses and Aaron in the wilderness. And the children of Israel said unto them, 'Oh, that we had died by the hand of the Lord in the land of Egypt, when we sat by the pots of meat and when we ate bread to the full! For you have brought us out into this wilderness, to kill this whole assembly with hunger." Exodus 16:2, 3.

Hunger is one of the strongest drives. Frequently, decisions regarding when to eat and how much to eat, are based solely on that drive. Eating three regular meals is not enough. Whenever and wherever the urge to eat manifests itself, most are apt to yield; eating whatever is available, whether there is really a biological need at the moment or not. A survey conducted by one of my students while I was a professor at Oakland University indicated that convenience, cost, and taste all take precedence over nutrition when selecting foods from vending machines. Far too often the results of uncontrolled appetite are manifested in bulging waistlines, a corpulence induced by the excessive intake of fats, sugars, and refined starches.

Most Americans have never suffered real hunger. I know I haven't. Oh, there have been times when my stomach grumbled louder and rumbled longer than I would have preferred, but there was always a refrigerator or convenience store nearby to disrupt the discomfort.

In developing countries like the Philippines the situation is quite different. Upwards of forty percent of the 84 million Filipinos go to bed hungry. This relentless hunger is repeated night after night after night. In large cities such as metro Manila, it is not uncommon to see five-year-olds, six-year-olds, and seven-year-olds, bellies protruding with the telltale signs of kwashiorkor, begging on the streets for a few pesos so that the gnaw of constant hunger can be temporarily stilled. Worldwide it is estimated that six million children under the age of five die from starvation every year.

We mustn't be too hard on the Israelites. Had we been there, in the same situation, what is to say that we too would not have longed for full bellies, gratified by the flesh pots of Egyptian delicacies. There they were, out in the middle of the desert, completely out of food and not a single grocery store within walking distance. The situation seemed as desperate as facing an impassable Red Sea had been. Notice carefully God's response to their cries. *"I will rain bread from heaven for you..., that I may test them, whether they will walk in My law or not."* Exodus 16:4.

In Exodus 15:26 — God had said, "Keep my laws and my statutes, and you will not get sick."

Then in Exodus 16:4, God said, "I've got a method. I've got a way to judge whether or not Israel will keep my commands."

How similar to the test given in the beginning in Eden when God said to Adam, "*Who told you that you were naked? Have you eaten of the tree that I told you not to eat of?*" Genesis 3:11.

Adam and Eve were tested on appetite to see whether or not they would fully obey God's word. Now as Israel began her journey to the Promised Land, God brought a similar test. "*I will rain bread from heaven **to prove** whether or not you will walk in my law.*"

Every Sunday, Monday, Tuesday, Wednesday, Thursday, and Friday morning, for the remainder of the journey, manna miraculously lay on the ground. If too much was gathered it stank, reinforcing the lesson that Israel needed to learn to trust God to provide daily food and not to worry about the future. Every Sabbath God provided another opportunity to trust in His word. No manna fell on the seventh day of the week, the Sabbath. But on Friday a double portion was to be gathered. Unlike the other days of the week, this extra manna was preserved for an additional 24 hours so that the Sabbath could be kept without needless work being performed on that day.

It may surprise some readers that manna was not the only food that God provided. Remember it wasn't something just to fill their tummies that Israel wanted. No they missed the meat they had eaten in Egypt. And so God granted that request also. "*And the Lord spake to Moses, saying, 'I have heard the complaints of the children of Israel.' Speak to them saying, 'At twilight you shall eat meat, and in the morning you shall be filled with bread. And you shall know that I am the Lord your God.*"

Thus it was that quails came up at evening and covered the camp..." Exodus 16:11–13.

Hmmm! Isn't that interesting? If God's ideal diet, given in Eden, is one that doesn't consist of meat, fowl, or fish, then what is He doing deliberately supplying birds to supplement the manna?

After so many years of slavery in Egypt, Israel had lost sight of many of God's commands to Abraham, Isaac, and Jacob. They had become lax in their obedience to God's law. Even though they had now been baptized in the Red Sea, they were not ready to inherit the Promised Land. There was still too much of "Egypt" in them. And so God took them on a circuitous detour through the desert, thereby giving them a chance to learn to trust in Him. And when they clamored for a meat based diet, He gave it to them. Yes, God gave them flesh in the wilderness, even though He knew it was not best for them.

What a marvelous God! Here I am, new in my Christian experience. I need to do a lot of growing before I reach God's lofty standards. In the process, God doesn't require me to make a fathom leap all at once. No, He says, "My child, here is my desire for you. However, at the moment you are a long, long way from that ideal. So here are some stepping stones to help you mature."

Thus begins my Christian experience. Day after day, I stumble. I fall. I blunder, and stumble all over again. But keeping my eyes on Jesus, I get up after each wrong. I get up and then take another step; moving forward towards the ideal that God has for me.

Then one day I do a self-evaluation. In health education we call this a process evaluation. I look back towards Egypt and see that indeed I have come a long way. I also realize that there are still some Egyptian relics that don't belong in my baggage. I know that these are hindering my Christian growth but I happen to like them. Besides these are not big sins. In fact I begin to think that maybe they shouldn't be called sins at all since so many other church members seem to be engaging in and enjoying them also. And so I begin to make excuses for my imperfect behavior. And I stop growing spiritually; having mistaken God's permission for his preferences.

Remember the story in Matthew 19, when the Pharisees came to Jesus and tried to trip him up on the law of divorce? *"Is it lawful for a man to put away his wife for every cause?"*

When Jesus answered by declaring the permanency of marriage they asked the question, *"Why did Moses then command to give a writing of divorcement, and to put her away."*

You'll recall Christ's answer, *"Moses, because of the hardness of your hearts suffered you to put your wives away, but from the beginning it was not so."* (Emphasis my own)

"From the beginning it was not so." It appears that over time, God allowed, or permitted, certain actions that did not fit in with His original plan. Why? Because of rebellion in the hearts of His people. But don't you think that as we get closer to Christ's second coming, God will empower His people to emulate His original ideal?

Take this subject of diet. Yes, in Leviticus 11 and Deuteronomy 14 God gave permission to eat the clean meats (without the fat and blood — See Leviticus 7:23–26). But from the beginning; from Creation, it was not so.

In the Exodus, God was leading Israel to the Promised Land. He was trying to develop in them the trust that Adam and Eve had forfeited. Realizing the Israelites had a lot of growing up to do, he provided quail in response to their clamoring. But only for a short time. Certainly by the time Israel reached Sinai, there daily fare consisted solely of manna and was free of flesh foods.

Complaining on the Borders of the Promised Land — Let's move ahead in time to Numbers 10. The Israelites were camped at the base of Mt. Sinai. It had been one year and two months since they left Egypt. For weeks, the pillar of fire by night and the cloud by day that had guided them, had remained stationary overhead. All of a sudden, on this bright sunny day, the cloud began to move. The command was given, — "Move northward." Canaan, the land of Promise, was less than a month away. Their journeyings in the harsh Wilderness of Sin were about to end. Oh, what excitement there must have been. What rejoicing! Perhaps Miriam and the ladies of Israel even dusted off the old tambourines and broke forth again in song and dance.

But old habits die hard. The complaining and blaming that began at the Red Sea fourteen months earlier, sprang up again. As if on cue the plaintive bellyaching choir raised its voice once more. The details are given in Numbers 11.

"Now the mixed multitude who were among them yielded to intense craving; (the King James Version says *"lusted") so the children of Israel also wept again and said, 'Who will give us meat to eat?*

We remember the fish, which we ate freely in Egypt; the cucumbers, the melons, the leeks, the onions, and the garlic;but now our whole being is dried up; there is nothing at all except this manna, before our eyes!"

"Manna, manna, manna! God, — that's all we get to eat! Sunday — manna. Monday — manna. Tuesday — manna. Wednesday — manna. Thursday — manna. Friday — manna. Even on Sabbath. All we ever get to eat is manna. We've been eating this stuff for the last year. And you know what, God? We are sick and tired of it!"

It reminds me of my canvassing days. While a sophomore at Columbia Union College in Takoma Park, Maryland, the Columbia Union initiated a program known as Campus Crusade Against Drugs (CCAD). Not only did it provide an opportunity to get *Listen* magazine and other anti-drug materials into the hands of high school youth, it also provided scholarship opportunities.

During the summer of 1972, programs were run in Pennsylvania, Maryland, Virginia, and New Jersey. In New Jersey, as many as 20 students from Columbia Union College, Garden State Academy, and Blue Mountain Academy concentrated their efforts in the resort towns along the Atlantic Coast.

A dear church member ran a summer boarding home on the island of Brigantine, just north of Atlantic City. Bless her heart, she agreed to rent the whole upstairs of the whitewashed two-story building to students in the CCAD campaign.

Now compared to the luxury hotels along Atlantic City's famed boardwalk, (today Donald Trump owns the ritziest hotels along that stretch), it was indeed modest. Yet for a group of academy and college students, nothing could beat spending the summer just one block from the beach, and getting paid for it?

Centrally situated on the second floor was a communal kitchen and dining area. Here we met for daily devotions along with our breakfast, which often consisted of cooked oatmeal and fruit.

Over the years I have come to enjoy oatmeal, especially on cold winter mornings. But back in the summer of 1972, cooked oatmeal had to be near the top of my list of least favorite foods. It probably stemmed from an aversion learned in childhood.

In my childhood home, cooked oatmeal was a staple of Sunday morning breakfasts. Whatever else might have been on the menu: pancakes, French toast, cornbread, white flour biscuits and chicken gravy (we were not vegetarians), mother just had to serve hot steaming bowls of oatmeal topped with sliced bananas and raisins—at the time two of my least favorite fruits. It was my belief that only the tablespoon or two of brown sugar generously sprinkled on top made it somewhat palatable. Fortunately Mom was kind enough to let me choose instead the sugar laden colder cereals, generally eaten dry.

Dry cereal, completely devoid of milk, juice, or even water, was a breakfast staple of mine during the preteen years. Whether it was Corn Flakes, Frosted Flakes, Wheaties, Cheerios, or even Shredded Wheat, it made no difference, the cereal was eaten as dry as could be. Mastication became a fine art that would have made Dr. Kellogg proud. I wonder how it was I never choked on those raw fibers.

Nor was devouring dry cereal, my only dietary quirk. For whatever reason, Mom had set menus, somewhat like the norm at an academy. I remember Monday nights we always ate white polished rice topped with margarine, cinnamon, and sugar. Tuesday was salmon casserole. Friday evenings there were always tuna salad sandwiches and soup. At least we got our omega-3's. And in those days we didn't need to worry about toxic levels of mercury in the fish.

Then there was Sabbath lunch. That was the one meal of the week that Dad took responsibility for preparing. Unfortunately Dad's culinary skills basically consisted of boiling eggs and slicing cheese. These also were on my top ten list of most disliked foods.

My dislike of hard boiled eggs and Velveeta cheese, coupled with my fondness for potato chips, led to some rather interesting, albeit bizarre creations. The ultimate epicurean delight was designed to obscure the obnoxious flavors of the above detested foods. It consisted of (No I am not making this up. I have two sisters who can attest to the veracity of the following.) a slice of bread spread with a generous layer of peanut butter. So far so good. Next came two slabs of cheese, followed by sliced hard boiled egg. (I warned you it was bizarre but it gets even worse. Keep reading.)

This was followed by slices of dill pickles over which a liberal amount of cinnamon and sugar was sprinkled. Then to make it palatable and crunchy, a layer of potato chips was inserted. Topped by another peanut butter smeared slice of bread, this "sandwich" was weekly Sabbath fare, until I went away to academy and decided it wasn't the wisest thing to create such a conglomeration in the presence of my peers.

So there I was in Brigantine, New Jersey in the summer of 1972, and morning after morning, I had to force myself to eat the detestable oatmeal. On a regular basis I voiced my displeasure.

"Why do we always have oatmeal for breakfast.?" This conference must really be poor if all they can afford to feed us is oatmeal."

After several days of listening to my griping, a colleague had heard enough. "Oatmeal, oatmeal, oatmeal! All we ever get to eat is oatmeal," Jim chanted. "Bill, you sound just like the Israelites complaining about the manna in the desert."

And I did. And it was probably in the same manner. Whatever legitimate excuses I thought I had, voicing such complaints tended to tear down and discourage others in the group rather than uplifting and encouraging them. And that's the problem with relentless complaining. It tears down, individually and corporately, rather than building up.

Look at what happened when a motley crew of hotheaded Israelites began hooting and hollering. Numbers 11 begins with, *"When the people complained, it displeased the Lord."*

Where Is God When the Future Is Dark? — You may not have thought about it before, but the Lord is not very pleased when we complain. Let me ask a question. Did the Israelites have legitimate concerns to complain about? You bet they did! In fact their fears and worries were much more legitimate than the petty things, like hard boiled eggs and oatmeal, that I have spent so much of my life complaining about.

Living as slaves under Pharaoh had not been the easiest life. But it was a lot more pleasant before Moses confronted Pharaoh with the ultimatum, *"Thus says the Lord God of Israel, 'Let my people go."*

Instead of finding freedom, the Israelites were flogged mercilessly. Instead of straw for bricks, they got a new task added to their job description. Yet production had to be maintained at previous levels. Downsizing is not something new. Its origins are based on enforced slave labor.

Next, catastrophes struck. The water supply became polluted with blood. Frogs jumped around the the bakeries and overran the restaurants. After that plaque had run its course and the land stank with the smell of putrefying amphibians, lice became problematic.

Have you ever noticed in your own life, how it seems that the harder you try to serve the Lord, the more troubles and problems come your way?

"Thus says the Lord," to the demons that surround you, "Let my people go."

Then Bam! Bam! Bam! In rapid succession comes problem, after problem, after problem! And in your agony you cry out, "God, where are you. Why don't you here my cries? Why don't you help me?"

In the dark periods of my life, out of an anguished heart, I too have uttered these sentiments. A few years ago, my family returned to the States after fulfilling our mission service. It seemed that everything in my life had all of a sudden gone downhill. I was struggling in my work. I was facing financial difficulties. We had just bought a house and were encountering a number of unexpected repairs. My daughter was having difficulties readjusting to life back in America. And it seemed that the prayer line to heaven had gone dead.

About this time, my younger sister, Nancy, shared with me the following passage from page 528 of <u>The Desire of Ages</u>. It is taken from the chapter on the resurrection of Lazarus. *"To all who are reaching out to feel the guiding hand of God, the moment of greatest discouragement is the time when divine help is nearest. They will look back with thankfulness upon the darkest part of their way. ... From every temptation and every trial He will bring them forth with firmer faith and a richer experience."*

The writer goes on to explain that if Christ had come immediately in response to the call that Lazarus was sick, Lazarus would not have died. But then Jesus would not have performed the miracle that was the greatest evidence of His divinity.

We need to come to the place in our lives where we trust God implicitly with the problems, and setbacks, and calamities, and yes, even deaths that He permits to take place. We need to have an all abiding faith that believes that the manna will fall just as surely today as it did yesterday, and that we do not need to store it up just in case there is a famine.

Had Israel known beyond a shadow of a doubt that within a few days they would be in Canaan, do you think they would have been complaining about the manna? I don't. The Bible says that shortly after entering Canaan, the manna stopped anyway. (See Joshua 5:11, 12)

Had Israel known the outcome of Jericho, and how God would fight their other Canaanite enemies with hailstones and hornets, do you think the ten spies would have been intimidated by the giants of the land? I don't.

Could it be that God sometimes permits unfathomable struggles in our lives so that He can manifest His power in delivering us?

"But God, that's not the route I want to take. I want the shortcut to Canaan. Oh yes, I want to follow you with all my heart, but only if the path is easy and the future is obstacle free."

No, I do not like the route God selects when it lurks with dangers and discouragement. I cringe and cower, and gripe and grumble about the pitfalls in the path. Oh, how desperately I need to realize and remember that God knows what he is doing, and in the end everything will turn out right.

The falling of the manna was a sandbox illustration of the capability of God to meet mankind's daily needs. How sad then that the very resource God gave for Israel's survival, became the source of her demise.

Numbers 11:10 — *"And the anger of the Lord was kindled greatly."*

Does God get angry? According to this text He does. One might even consider that the wording indicates He was furious.

What makes God angry?

When His people have had demonstration after demonstration of His watch care and protection, when miracle after miracle has been performed in their behalf, and they still refuse to trust Him but rather lust after the treasures and pleasures of Egypt. This is a mockery to God and He doesn't take it lightly.

Yet despite their cravings for the things of Egypt, despite their desire for that which the world offered, God still answered Israel's prayers. *"You shall not eat flesh one day, nor two days, nor five days, neither 10 days, nor 20 days, but even a whole month, until it comes out at your nostrils and is loathsome to you."*

Moses was astonished. He could not believe what he was hearing. Meat to feed the whole camp for a month? Perhaps he needed to remind God that the Israelites numbered 600,000 footmen plus women and children. It was going to take a lot of hamburger and they hadn't come across any local Wendy's or MacDonald's. Where was all this meat coming from?

So he asked, *"Shall flocks and herds be slaughtered for them? Or shall all the fish of the sea be gathered together for them, to provide enough for them?"*

It is within this context that we find an oft quoted text, *"Has the Lord's arm been shortened? Now you will see whether what I say will happen to you or not."*

We use this passage when we want to assure ourselves that nothing is too difficult for God to accomplish. But the context has God uttering these words at a time when He is distraught with His people. The lesson here is that one needs to be careful in what he or she demands from the Lord. You just may get what you ask for; even though it is not in your best interest.

Verse 31 — "Now *a wind went out from the Lord, and it brought quail from the sea, and left them fluttering near the camp, about a day's journey on this side, and about a day's journey on the other side, all around the camp, and about two cubits above the surface of the ground.*

How far is a day's journey? One mile? Two miles? Ten miles? In Hong Kong, I conducted a running clinic. Many in the clinic were able to finish a marathon (approximately 26 miles or 42 kilometers) in less than five hours. So how far is a day's journey?

Considering the size of the Israelite camp, including children, pregnant women, their cattle and belongings, let's be ultra-conservative and say that a day's journey was only a mile or 1.6 kilometers. There, encompassing the camp in every direction, as far as the eye could see were quail flying around at waist level.

This was one catch the Israelites were not going to let slip away. Chores were forgotten. Their tiredness dissipated. Even the complaining stopped as the people focused on cramming the larders with bird food. Yes, a diet of quail was nothing but bird food compared to the bread of heaven with which God had been feeding them.

And the people stayed up all that day, all night, and all the next day, and gathered the quail.

Talk about marathons. This was a non-stop, 36-hour, all you can grab, hunt.

"He that gathered least gathered 10 homers."

Now what's a *"homer?"* The only "homer" that I know of is when a baseball player hits the ball out of the park and circles the bases before crossing home plate. That's a homer. But being sure that baseball was not played in Biblical times, I went to the dictionary. There I learned that a homer is ten bushels. So he who gathered least, gathered 100 bushels. That's a lot of quail by any standard. Certainly more than enough for a gluttonous orgy.

It was as if the whole camp had been starving for days. There were quail burgers, quail steaks, quail salad, and quail you-name-it. In whatever form or shape they could eat it, the Israelites gorged themselves on quail.

But in the midst of the feast, ptomaine poisoning broke out. Thousands died with undigested quail still in their mouths. And Numbers 11 ends with a great funeral service.

How sad. Yet it isn't the premature and unnecessary deaths that make this story so sad. There are other texts of Scripture where large numbers of God's people died. What makes these verses so sad is the time frame within which they occurred.

Just two chapters later, the Bible relates the story of the spies entering Canaan to scout out the land. You see, the grumbling, the griping, the complaining — the deaths in Numbers 11, occurred just before Israel reached the Promised Land.

Relevance of the Manna for Seventh-day Adventists — "Okay," you say. "All of this has been a nice story, albeit with a sad ending. But how does it relate to me today? What relevance does it have in a book on the history of the Adventist health message?"

Remember in I Corinthians 10, Paul compares the Exodus to the experience of God's people living in the last days. *"Moreover, brethren, I do not want you to be unaware that all our fathers were under the cloud, all passed through the sea,*

And were all baptized into Moses in the cloud and in the sea,

All ate the same spiritual food,

And all drink the same spiritual drink. For they drank of that spiritual Rock that followed them, and that Rock was Christ.

But with most of them God was not well pleased, for their bodies were scattered in the wilderness.

Now these things were written for our examples, to the intent that we should not lust after evil things, as they also lusted."

The symbolism here is rich. Egypt represents the world—apostasy—a lusting after things that are contrary to God's will.

Israel is symbolic of God's people living in the last days of earth's history.

Canaan depicts the heavenly Canaan.

Israel's journey from Egyptian bondage to the Promised Land is illustrative of our deliverance from sin and the trials and obstacles along the pathway to heaven.

The crossing of the Red Sea represents baptism.

The manna shows the need for daily feeding on the living Word of God.

The story of Israel's journey to the Promised Land makes one thing clear. The closer I get to the Promised Land, the less of Egypt should be in my life. When in Exodus 16, Israel first expressed cravings for the Egyptian diet, it was shortly after her Red Sea "baptismal" experience. The Israelites were like babes and had much to learn.

In Christianity, baptism represents a public declaration of a born-again decision. But remember, at the time of baptism, a person is still a baby in regards to his or her Christian experience. There is a lot of growing that needs to take place before a Christ-like character has developed. This growth the Bible refers to as sanctification.

This is why in Matthew 28, Jesus commands that following baptism, the church must teach and instruct new believers. This aspect of the gospel commission must not be neglected. The church must have ongoing Bible study classes to ground newly baptized members in the fullness of the doctrines of Jesus Christ. Church members must be patient with new believers in their growing. There will be some stumbling and falling along the way as God tries to weed the roots of Egypt out of their lives. During these trying times, they especially need the special encouragement and love of their older brothers and sisters in Christ.

Eventually all born-again Christians arrive at Sinai. From that point onwards, God expects things to be different in our lives.

For it is in those miniature Sinais that God reveals His will fully. At Sinai, He thunders his holy Ten Commandments. At Sinai, He reveals the total plan of salvation in the sanctuary: justification, sanctification, and glorification. It is at Sinai that the believer becomes grounded in sound doctrine. At Sinai, anything that smacks of an Egyptian lifestyle is removed, for at Sinai mankind is standing on holy ground. It is here that God declares, "You shall be holy, for I am holy."

Israel camped at the foot of Sinai for almost one and a half years. God was patient with them. He gave them time to get to know Him. He was preparing them for entrance into Canaan.

Then one day, in the middle of Numbers 10, the cloud started moving northward. This was the signal for Israel to strike camp and move forward. Their journeying in the desert was about to end. Israel was almost home. Kadesh-Barnea, on the border of the Promised Land, was only eleven days away.

Notice an interesting parallel. Three days after the crossing of the Red Sea, Israel began complaining. And three days after leaving Sinai, Israel again began complaining. It seems that even after a year and a half at Sinai, the Israelites were no more prepared to trust God than when they had crossed the Red Sea. And because they had never learned to trust God with something as simple as appetite, they were totally unprepared to trust Him when confronted with the giants that were soon to come into their lives.

There is more to the health message than just learning how to avert illness and premature death. If in our zeal we are simply promoting a lifestyle that adds up to a decade of additional life, we are only making healthier sinners. While avoiding sickness and living longer are important benefits, if this is all that others see in our health message, then we have failed miserably in its proclamation.

I believe that the ultimate reason God has given the Seventh-day Adventist Church a health reform message is to prepare a people to enter the heavenly Promised Land. Though this message entails more than diet, the Bible reveals that food is often used as a test to determine whether God's people will obey Him or not.

Adam and Eve lost paradise because of a wrong choice regarding their diet.

Esau sold his birthright for a pot of lentil stew.

The widow of Zapparoth, down to her last morsel before starvation, passed the test and God honored her faith by miraculously providing for her day after day.

Jesus' first temptation in the wilderness was to "turn stones into bread."

And the manna of the Exodus stank if hoarded in violation of God's commands.

Uncontrolled appetite — such a small matter in the overall scheme of things. Certainly it is a much, much less grievous sin than murder, or adultery, or stealing, or loss of temper, or taking God's name in vain. Yet, I would suggest that the giving of the manna teaches that as long as I clamor after the diet of the world, I will never learn to trust God in other areas of my life.

I would also suggest that my food choices indicate whether my focus is on heaven or whether with forlorn gaze I am still looking backwards towards Egypt. My purpose here is not to specify in detail what a person should eat and drink, and what one shouldn't. Often even the best choices are mitigated by availability, economics, extent of nutritional knowledge, and other factors.

But God has clearly revealed that the diet of choice for His people is the one that He gave in the beginning. It was the best for man at creation and it still will provide the best health for God's people living in the 21st century. Genesis 1:29, "See, *I have given you every herb that yields seed which is on the face of all the earth, and every tree whose fruit yields seed; to you it shall be for food.*"

God went on to say that man could eat liberally of this diet. Genesis 2:16, "*Of every tree of the garden you may freely eat.*"

After Adam and Eve sinned, vegetables were added to the menu. Genesis 3:18, "*You shall eat the herb of the field.*"

As we get nearer and nearer to our heavenly home, shouldn't we strive to make this diet of fruits, grains, nuts, vegetables, and seeds, our predominant diet? Shouldn't we now be conditioning our taste buds and stomachs to the diet of heaven so that when we get there we will be accustomed to it?

The promise of Exodus 15:26, "*I will put none of these diseases upon you,*" is still valid today. But as long as His children are clamoring for the diet of Egypt, God can neither pour out the physical healing, nor the spiritual blessings that He would like to.

Dear Reader, my prayer is that God will give you an appetite for the diet of heaven, so that you might be a fit, sturdy vessel that God can use for the proclamation of the gospel.

Let's not fail the test as did Israel. Remember the journey is almost over. We are standing on the very borders of the Promised Land. Jesus will soon return.

Now is the time to be strong. Now is the time to have courage. Now is the time to trust God in body, mind, and soul. Now is the time to lift up your head and rejoice because …

Hallelujah! We are almost home!

Chapter 12

THE SPIRIT OF CALEB

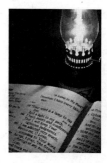

...Behold, the Lord has kept me alive, as He said, these forty-five years, ... And now, here I am this day, eighty-five years old.

As yet I am as strong this day as on the day Moses sent me; just as my strength was then, so now is my strength for war, both for going out and coming in.

Now therefore give me this mountain.
Joshua 14:10–12

Breaking the pattern of the previous chapters, I am going to start the final chapter with a quiz, rather than a story. You'll have to forgive me but my teaching background is manifesting itself. So is a page from my childhood in which Sabbath afternoons were often filled playing Bible games or quizzes.

I must warn you ahead of time that even though this is a short quiz, it is not an easy one. Okay, ready? Here are the first three questions.

1. Who was Shammua?

2. Who was Shaphat?

3. Who was Sethur?

Not doing so well? I warned you it might be a bit difficult. Well try number four.

4. Who was Gaddiel?

I don't think question five gets any easier.

5. Who was Ammiel?

Perhaps a few clues will help. All of the above were males. They were contemporaries. They were all leaders. They were all eyewitnesses of many miracles. They all played an important role in the Old Testament.

Still completely in the dark? Sorry, but you will have to read on a bit further to find the answers.

When I first gave a vesper series on the reasons for the Adventist health message, I entitled the final presentation, "Vegeburgers and Righteousness by Faith." In it I quoted rather extensively from the Spirit of Prophecy. There were quotations such as:

"It is as truly a sin to violate the laws of our being as it is to break the ten commandments. To do either is to break God's laws." Christian Temperance and Bible Hygiene, 53.

"Our first duty, one which we owe to God, to ourselves, and to our fellow men, is to obey the laws of God, which include the laws of health." Testimonies, Vol.3, 164–165.

"It is not possible for us to glorify God while living in violation of the laws of life." The Health Reformer, 181.

"It is just as much sin to violate the laws of our being as to break one of the ten commandments. We cannot love the Lord with all our heart, mind, soul, and strength while we are loving our appetites, our tastes, a great deal better than we love the Lord." Testimonies, Vol.2, 70.

"But those who are slaves to appetite will fail in perfecting Christian character.... As we near the close of time, Satan's temptation to indulge the appetite will be more powerful and more difficult to overcome." Testimonies, Vol.3, 491–492.

Now I believe that there is a strong connection between our physical condition and spiritual well-being. Paul pleads in Romans 12:1, *"I beseech you therefore brethren, by the mercies of God, that you present your bodies, a living sacrifice, holy, acceptable to God."*

Yet to quote Spirit of Prophecy writings, reference after reference after reference, proved to be a misappropriation of these wonderful truths. Often it felt as if I were using a hammer rather than a potter's wheel. Rather than evolving as a beautiful masterpiece, the health message was crumbling into a pile of shattered vessels.

One Sabbath morning in Hong Kong, while teaching a lesson on the manna and the ensuing disappointment at Kadesh-Barnea, the Lord impressed me with insights I had never seen before. Many of those insights were shared in the previous chapter. Additional study and contemplation led to the following discoveries—discoveries which give balance to the proclamation of our health message.

So who were those five men in the quiz — Shammua, Shaphat, Sethur, Gaddiel, and Ammiel?

Actually they were members of a larger group. Twelve to be exact. They were all spies, sent to search out the enemy's cities, and fortresses. Their assignment was to bring back a report on their foes' strengths and weaknesses Other members of the scouting party had names that were just as obscure — Nahbi, Igal, Ahiman, Talmai, and Geuel.

But the two remaining spies? Ah, they are household names to every Bible student — Caleb and Joshua.

Yes, the names of all twelve spies are recorded in the thirteenth chapter of Numbers. All were assigned to the Canaan search party because they were proven leaders in their tribes. They were men who had shouldered responsibility. They were men whom Moses felt he could depend upon.

Yet today, only two are remembered — Caleb and Joshua. The other ten are never again mentioned in Scripture. Upon returning from their spy mission, they never again set foot within the Promised Land. And it is likely that due to their lack of faith, they will never set foot in the heavenly Canaan either.

What made the difference between Caleb and Joshua, and the other ten? Twelve men were sent on an errand. They saw the same things, ate the same food, wandered the same byways, encountered the same difficulties, came face-to-face with the same giants. Yet ten of them cowered in fear. Ten shrank from confronting the challenges ahead. Ten opted for the path of least resistance and saw their futures end in obscurity and oblivion. Except for a single mention in Numbers 13, even their names are totally forgotten.

Attitude Makes the Difference — A multitude of 600,000 men, plus women and children, left Egypt for the Promised Land. Yet out of that horde, Caleb and Joshua were the only adults who made it. Therefore, don't you think it behooves us to dig deeply to discover what it was that made the difference in their lives?

I believe the answer is tucked away in Numbers 14:24. *"But My servant Caleb, because he has a different spirit in him, and has followed me fully, I will bring into the land where he went; and his descendants shall inherit it."*

Caleb — an example of those who will finally enter the heavenly Canaan — made it into the earthly Canaan, because he had *a different spirit within him*.

While others doubted, Caleb's faith held firm.

When others voiced doom and gloom, Caleb proclaimed valor and victory.

Where others saw monumental giants blocking the way, Caleb envisioned towering monuments of conquest.

When others whined and complained in discouragement and despair, Caleb rebuked them with words of faith in the power of God to overcome all of life's problems and difficulties.

"Because my servant Caleb has a different spirit within him, I will bring him into the land where he went!" This different spirit, or attitude, can be seen operating in three aspects of Caleb's life: 1) The way Caleb reacted to people

who caused him problems and difficulties. 2) The way Caleb reacted when others were promoted ahead of him. 3) The way Caleb responded to God's commands.

The first record of Caleb is in Numbers 13 where he is listed with the other spies. "So *Moses sent them from the Wilderness of Paran according to the command of the Lord, all of them men who were heads of the children of Israel. Now these were their names:... From the tribe of Judah, Caleb the son of Jephunneh.*"

As a matter of fact, out of the twelve spies, the only one whom the Bible mentions in earlier passages is Joshua. In Exodus 24, when Moses climbed Mt. Sinai to receive the ten commandments, Joshua went part of the way with him. In Exodus 33:11, Joshua is referred to as the servant of Moses as he accompanied him to the tabernacle. Perhaps he was his press secretary or aide-de-camp. But Caleb, on the other hand, isn't mentioned at all until the Israelites were about to enter the Promised Land.

The experience of the Israelites turning back into the desert should never have been written. It should not have been part of the Bible story. From the beginning of the Exodus, God had promised the Israelites that he would bring them into the land of their fathers, Abraham, Isaac, and Jacob. Now, they were almost there. They were almost home.

Then why the rebellion in chapter 11 over such a small item as food? Or was it really such a small matter after all? Wasn't manna the diet that God had chosen specifically for them? He could have have just as easily provided them with hamburgers, French fries, and milk shakes. In the manna, God gave to Israel the best diet possible. After eating it for more than a year there was "not one feeble person among them." In lusting after the foods the world was eating, the Israelites were actually revolting against God's plan for their lives.

The SAD Diet — Are we really any different from them? Don't we also crave the Egyptian diet; the diet that the world clamors for? Ask yourself the question, "Is there a difference between the food choices I make, and the choices made by my non-SDA neighbors and friends?"

Next time you're in the checkout line at the supermarket, compare the contents of your cart with that of the customer ahead of you. Is there a noticeable difference in the foods selected? If we are seeking to eat God's prescribed diet, there should be.

Could it be that God's people today are opting for the Standard American Diet (SAD) of the world, when we should be promoting the Standard Diet of Adventists (SDA) as given by God in Genesis 1:29 and 3:18?

The medical literature makes it clear that the primary diseases that are killing us, are caused by bad lifestyle habits, especially unhealthy diets. The Standard American Diet is loaded with saturated fat, cholesterol, sugar, and refined carbohydrates washed down with copious quantities of cola, soft drinks, coffee, and tea.

Western civilization is ravaged by heart disease, cancer, and strokes. Type II diabetes has reached epidemic proportions. Alzheimer's has become one of the top 10 killer's in America. More than 60% of Americans have an overweight problem. America is a sick nation and getting sicker despite the highest expenditure of any nation in the world on health care. As Dr. George Malkmus of Hallelujah Acres likes to put it, "We do not have a health care system in this country, we have a sick care system. And Americans are getting sicker by the minute."[1]

But these dietary induced illnesses are not limited solely to a decadent America. They have become global in impact. While a graduate student at Loma Linda in the 1980's I was interested in some of the research being done in Japan since it had the highest life expectancy in the world. Researchers were intrigued by the fact that here was an industrialized nation where heart disease was extremely low. How things have changed! Even though Japan continues to have the highest life expectancy rates, heart disease is in epidemic proportions and has become one of the top three killers in Japan.

When in 1993, I became director of Health Promotion and Wellness at the Hong Kong Adventist Hospital, I was surprised to learn that the three leading killers in Hong Kong were cancer, heart disease, and stroke. Then in 2000, my family and I moved to the Philippines, a developing country faced with the contagious diseases common in the tropics. I began to gather information on the country's morbidity and mortality profile. As expected, I found that the most prevalent disease was an infectious one, namely pneumonia. But I was astonished to learn that heart disease had become the Philippines number one killer.

Around the world, via its fast food industry and tobacco sales, American industries are exporting disease and death to developed and developing countries alike. And even though Adventists live longer, there isn't much difference between the diseases that we are dying from and those that the rest of the world are dying from. It's just that we postpone them a bit longer. Somehow, this doesn't seem quite right. Shouldn't serving God give us some sort of immunity from the ravages of sin, including those pathogens that strike directly at our physical well-being? Yet if we choose to live like the world, and if we choose to eat like the world; then we will get sick and die like the world.

God wants His children to be healthy. The promise of Exodus 15:26, *"If you will keep my commandments and obey my statutes, I will put none of these diseases upon you,"* is just as much for modern Israel as it was for the ancient Jews. That is a major reason why from its very inception, He gave Seventh-day Adventists a message of health. But I cannot claim the promises while continuing to abuse my body through eating the wrong foods, avoiding daily physical exercise, neglecting adequate sleep, being intemperate, and walking about with the wrong spirit or attitude.

Caleb — Going Against the Majority — When the spies went into Canaan, all twelve came back with a glowing report of the goodness of the land. They returned with baskets brimming with figs and pomegranates. They bore clusters of grapes so enormous that they had to be carried on a staff between two men. Imagine how appealing the sight of that food must have been to people who just weeks earlier had been complaining about their diet.

But all this was lost sight of because of the giants in the land.

And now at the crucial moment, for the first time Caleb stepped forward into the annals of Biblical history. He could not believe what he was hearing. After 40 days in the land flowing with milk and honey, all that his comrades focused on was the perceived threat posed by the Amalekites, the Hittites, the Jebusites, the Amorites, and Canaanites; all avowed enemies of the God of Abraham, Isaac, and Jacob.

In desperation Caleb cried out, *"Let us go up at once, and possess it; for we are able to overcome it."*

Joshua then joined him in trying to stop the rapidly growing discontent. In one last futile effort they rent their clothes and pled with their compatriots not to rebel against God.

"The Lord is with us; Fear them not!" they cried in vain.

In response the whole congregation picked up stones. Had God not intervened, Joshua and Caleb would have lost their lives.

The Bible account then records two of the saddest verses in all of Scripture — Numbers 14:22, 23. *"Because all these men who have seen My glory and the signs which I did in Egypt and in the wilderness, and have put Me to the test now these ten times, and have not heeded my voice,* **they certainly will not see the land** *which I swore to their fathers, nor shall any of those who rejected Me see it."*

"They certainly will not see the land." So close to home; yet so very very far away. Their hopes, their dreams, the very reason for their journey — all of it shattered because of an ability to trust in the power of an Almighty God to perform what He had promised.

Back Into the Wilderness — So instead of celebrating in their new home, the children of Israel found themselves making a 180 degree turnabout. For 38 more years they wandered as nomads. The harshness of the desert became their permanent lot. And the detested manna was all they got to eat, until one by one they passed away into oblivion, their carcasses buried in the sand of the Wilderness of Sin.

How sad! How tragic! How fraught with warnings to us "upon whom the ends of the world are come."

It is within the context of this tragedy that the nobility of Caleb emerged. For Caleb too had to turn around and head back into the harsh, unforgiving wilderness.

What is the desert like? For those living in moderate temperature zones or in tropical climates it is hard to comprehend. Much of southern California, where we lived for 14 years, is desert. Periodically we would visit Joshua Tree National Park in the Mojave Desert, east of Palm Springs, California. Within its confines, the magnitude of its barrenness and harshness would strike us. Deserts are hot, dry, and unbearable. Their sandy floors sustain only sparse clumps of the hardiest grasses and shrubs. Animal life is limited to rodents, toads, snakes, and predators such as coyotes and foxes. Cacti, with sharp spines, provide limited shelter and food. Rainfall amounts to only a few centimeters per year. Despite the unbearable daytime heat, temperatures can plummet to near freezing after sundown. Deserts are indeed harsh environments with numerous challenges for survival.

As Israel was compelled to endure her plight, God went back into the wilderness with her. During the day, the cloud provided respite from the heat. During the night, that same cloud provided light and warmth. It was a daily testimony that the God they had rebelled against, was a God they could still rely upon. And day by day, He continued to remind them of His power to sustain by continuing to supply them with manna.

During those 38 years, Caleb wandered in obscurity. He suffered just like the other Israelites, through no fault of his own. What thoughts must have gone through his head? I know the thoughts that would have gone through mine.

"God, this is unfair. I wasn't the one who grumbled and complained and rebelled. No, in case you forgot God, I was the one who was willing to risk death to defend your name. And now you put me through this? God, you're not being fair. Why should I have to suffer because of these stupid ungrateful gripers who do nothing but complain all day any way?" That's what Bill Andress would have been tempted to think for all those years. But not Caleb.

Look at Numbers 14:24 again. — *My servant Caleb had a different spirit within him.* Caleb's faith in the omniscience of God was so strong that difficulties perpetrated by his peers could not shake it. When the actions of others caused troubles in his own life, he did not retaliate, but rather maintained an attitude of *"all things work together for good to them that love the Lord."*

That same spirit would keep us from getting angry at our spouses, our kids, our co-workers, the driver who cuts us off, the person who spreads malicious gossip behind our backs. Oh, how desperately each of us needs the humble spirit of Caleb, because it is the spirit of Christ.

But that's not the only way in which a different spirit, or attitude, was manifested in Caleb. After Numbers 14, for the next 45 years of his life, the Bible is virtually silent regarding Caleb. Those few verses that do mention him always include Joshua in the same passage. And it is always Joshua, not Caleb, who is ascending to a position of preeminence. In Numbers 27, Joshua is promoted to commander-in-chief of the armies of Israel. In Numbers 34, along with Eliezar the priest, he is given charge of divvying up the land of Canaan. In Deuteronomy 1, it is Joshua who is appointed as Moses' successor. It is Joshua who leads Israel across the Jordan into the Promised Land. And it is Joshua who gets the glory at the battle of Jericho.

Again Caleb is bypassed. If I had been Caleb, my thinking would have gone something like this. "Why

192 • Adventist Heritage of Health

should Joshua get all the promotions? I was just as faithful. I have equal leadership abilities. If for no other reason, I should be selected over him because I am older
and therefore more mature and experienced. As a matter
of fact, if you study the historical record carefully, you
will find in Numbers 13:30 that it was I, not Joshua, who
first sought to calm the mob when the other spies brought
back a report of fear and trepidation. So God, how come
it is Joshua who gets all the glory, all the attention, and
all the promotions?"

Isn't this how we tend to react when a colleague gets
promoted ahead of us, or someone is given a reward that
we think we are more qualified to receive. But not Caleb.

My servant Caleb had a different spirit within him.

You see, Caleb was focused on a much larger goal, an
uncompleted task. It was an undertaking of gigantic proportions. He didn't have time to be sidetracked by petty
distractions or get caught up in egoistic power struggles.

After years of aimless meandering in the desert, the
nation of Israel finally did settle into Canaan. Left behind
was a Sinai peninsula littered with the graves of those 20-
years and older who had demonstrated a lack of faith at
Kadesh-Barnea. Included among the tombs were those of
Miriam, and Aaron. Even Moses, who at one time pleaded
with God to remove his name from the Book of Life if the
children of Israel could not inherit the Promised Land,
had to face death on the wrong side of the Jordan. How
sad, how heart rending. Of the hundreds of thousands of
adults who left Egypt, only Joshua and Caleb realized the
fulfillment of their dreams.

Caleb was not satisfied to simply take up residency in
Canaan. No, there was unfinished business that needed
to be taken care of. Years earlier he had seen his compatriots cower in fear of the giants stalking the land. As
family members and friends died in the Wilderness of
Sin he couldn't help but recognize that it was all because
of their lack of faith in God's power to deal with those
giants. Caleb had a score to settle. Those giants had to

be destroyed! Until that happened there was always the possibility that the current generation of Israelites would also tremble in fear and flee in their presence.

Oh, that we would be like Caleb! A man not threatened by giants. A man not discouraged by the obstacles in his life. A man secure in his faith in God. A man who rather than seeking retirement, remained on the battlefield until every enemy of the Lord was defeated.

Sometimes it helps to give names to the giants that block our path. By giving them names, the obstacles become more clearly defined and we are able to focus better. Caleb gave names to his giants, — Ahiman, Sheihai and Talmai — all three sons of Anak, father of the Anakims, one of the tribes of "great and tall men" in the land of Canaan.

And then he set out to destroy those giants.

Then the children of Judah came unto Joshua in Gilgal. And Caleb the son of Jephunah, the Kenezite said to him, . . .

The Lord has kept me alive, as He said, these forty-five years, ever since the Lord spoke this word to Moses while Israel wandered in the wilderness; and now, here I am this day eighty-five years old.

As yet I am as strong this day as on the day Moses sent me; just as my strength was then, so now is my strength for war, both for going out and coming in.

Now therefore give me this mountain of which the Lord spoke in that day; for you heard in that day how the Anakim were there, and that the cities were great and fortified. It may be that the Lord will be with me, and I shall be able to drive them out as the Lord said." Joshua 14:6, 10–12.

What invincible faith! What courage! What a testimony of obedience to God's statutes and commandments. Did you catch it? At the age of 85, Caleb proclaimed that he was just as strong as he had been when he was 40-years-old.

Most fear the aging process because it is seen as a time of demise. Senior citizens are viewed as hapless, helpless, hopeless humans who are sliding down a slippery slope to their sepulchers. But Caleb's testimony validates that it doesn't have to be this way. Through obedience Caleb experienced the fulfillment of the promises of God. *"If you will keep all my statutes, I will put none of these diseases upon you which I have brought upon the Egyptians"* and *"I will prolong your days upon the earth."*

In a previous chapter, I highlighted the accomplishments of Hulda Crooks in her eighties and nineties. A few years after her exploits on Mt. Fuji, I had the privilege of assisting in testing another 80-year-old on the treadmill. Her name was Mavis Lindgren. Like Hulda, Mavis had been sickly in her teens and early adult life. And what was true for Hulda, also was true for Mavis. Exercise and adherence to a Genesis 1:29 diet, turned her life around.

She ran her first marathon at the youthful age of sixty. During the next ten years she completed five marathons a year. When I first met her she was preparing to run her 51st. The treadmill test measured the ability of her body to utilize oxygen on the cellular level. Results indicated she had the fitness level of the average college age girl. No wonder that news reporters referred to her as "Amazing Mavis."

Recently the prestigious *National Geographic* ran a cover story on longevity.[2] One of three groups featured were Seventh-day Adventists living in Loma Linda. Individuals in their 100's, who were still actively pursuing a life similar to what they had enjoyed when they had been 40 years younger, were interviewed. The article pointed out that the critical factor in determining longevity is not genetics, but lifestyle.

Still, as I have asserted several times in this book, if all the Adventist health message can offer is a few more years on planet earth, then we have completely missed what it is all about. The Adventist health message is a doctrine designed to teach people how to add eternity to their lives. It needs to be presented as a message that will enable its adherers to live forever in an earth made new, where there is no more pain, suffering, sadness, disease, or death. In its purity it can never be taught without an emphasis on the third characteristic of the "spirit of Caleb" and that is, *"Caleb wholly followed the Lord."* Numbers 14:24.

Really it's as simple as that. When God proclaimed the Ten Commandments, Caleb simply said, "I will follow and obey."

When God gave a plain diet of daily manna, Caleb didn't lust after the rich delicacies of Egypt.

When God said, "I have prepared for you a land of milk and honey," Caleb was not intimidated by the giants that needed to be driven out.

When God said, "Head back into the desert for 38 more years," Caleb went — not understanding the whys and wherefores, but believing the safest path for his life was the one that followed God's leadings.

And by the time God finally allowed Caleb to receive as his inheritance, any portion of the Promised Land that his heart desired, he had developed such a strong confidence in His Lord and Savior that he asked for the privilege of having the glory of defeating the very giants that had delayed the fulfillment of his dreams for forty-five years.

Not only did Caleb drive out those giants — Sheshai, Ahiman, and Talmai, the sons of Anak, — but he conquered their fortress, Hebron as well. Hebron then became the inheritance of Caleb, and "the *land had rest from war.*"

Later, Hebron was ceded to the Levites and became a city of refuge. Here is another message of hope for those who are struggling with their own fearful giants. God can take that which is too big for you and threatens to destroy you, and change it into a fortification of refuge—a place that is safe and secure.

Oh, that God's people today would manifest the spirit of Caleb! It is a sprit that is not bothered by the vicissitudes of life. It is a spirit that rejoices in the successes and sympathizes with the disappointments of those around us. It is a spirit that fights for right and turns enemy bastions into safe havens for God's people.

Caleb was able to accomplish what he did because he purposed to "follow the Lord wholly." And it is this purpose that provides a solid foundation for the Adventist message of hope and healing.

In these final days of earth's history, God is preparing a people who will march victoriously into the Promised Land. Like Caleb, they will follow the Lord wholly, — not just spiritually; not just intellectually, — but physically as well. They will be a people in whom the image of God has been completely restored.

The year was 1973. Most Americans old enough to remember, can recall the long waits at gasoline pumps as they suffered through weeks of "oil shock." I was a student missionary in Osaka, Japan at the time. The effects of the heightened tensions in the Middle East were especially significant since Japan was importing almost 100% of its oil from that region. There were controlled power outages at night, escalating prices in the supermarkets, and the hoarding of such basic essentials as toilet paper.

Into the wee hours of the morning, my roommates and I talked about never returning to the United States of America to complete our college degrees, so sure were we that Jesus would return to earth before our year in Japan was finished. Our English as a Second Language students began attending our Bible classes in ever increasing numbers. They were eager to know what the Bible had to say about world events that were unfurling. From August 1973 to the following August, the SDA language schools in Japan had one of their highest baptismal rates ever. We student missionaries had a sense that it was because some droplets from the latter rain were beginning to fall.

Now it is 34 years later. Jesus has not returned. His people are still wandering in this desolate, harsh, wilderness of sin. Friends, family members, loved ones have died on the wrong side of the Jordan. Sometimes the road gets pretty discouraging and all we can see up ahead are the giant sons of Anak. We start feeling like grasshoppers and are tempted to surrender the fight. But beloved, do not give up! Maintain the unwavering spirit of Caleb. Hold firm to the promises of God. He wants you to have victory. He will empower you to conquer in the name of Jesus Christ.

Return with me to the challenge that Moses gave to Israel in his farewell address. It was an address that Joshua repeated to the Israelites once they were settled in the Promised Land. Joshua placed half the camp on Mt. Gerizim and half the camp on Mt. Ebal. Between the two mountains lay the Vale of Shechem, the best watered valley in central Palestine. And from there Joshua redelivered the farewell speech that Moses had made forty years earlier as recorded in Deuteronomy chapters 27–31.[3] In it he reminded Israel of the great things God would do for them if they would but commit to obeying Him fully.

It is a message that prepared ancient Israel to inherit the Land of Promise and it is a message that will prepare you, dear reader, to inherit the heavenly kingdom.

"If you diligently obey the voice of the Lord your God, to observe carefully all His commandments, that I command you today, that the Lord your God will set you high above all nations of the earth....

And the Lord shall make you the head and not the tail; you shall be above only, and not be beneath, if you heed the commandments of the Lord your God, and are careful to observe them....

Therefore keep the words of this covenant, and do them, that you may prosper in all that you do...." Deuteronomy 28:1; 28:13, 29:9.

You are part of that special group that God wants to bring into the heavenly Canaan. During the journey He has promised to heal your diseases[4] and cause you to mount up with eagle's wings.[5] He wants to make you an example to the world of what can be accomplished through the most humble life that is committed to Him. He wishes above all things that *"you may prosper and be in health, even as your soul prospers."*

Today, God sets forth the same challenge to godliness that He declared through Moses and Joshua nearly 4,000 years ago, *"I have set before you life and death, blessing and cursing: therefore **choose life,** that both you and your descendants may live:*

That you may love the Lord your God, and that you may obey His voice, and that you may cling to Him: for He is your life, and the length of your days."

This proclamation is the essence of the Adventist Heritage of Health, Hope, and Healing —

Therefore Choose Life!

APPENDIX

Some Biblical Principles for a Healthy Lifestyle	
Eat only that which is good.	Isa. 55:2; Gen. 3:29
Avoid overeating and gluttony.	Deut. 21:20; Phil. 3:19
Avoid eating empty calorie foods.	Prov. 23:1-3
Eat for strength and not self gratification.	Eccles.10:17
Eat at regular times, avoiding in-between meal snacks.	Eccles. 3:1
Balance your life with exercise and rest.	Exod. 20:9,10; Ps. 127:2; Eccles. 5:12
Drink adequate water daily (at least 8 glasses).	Rev. 22:17
Be temperate and moderate in your habits of life.	I Cor. 9:25; Phil. 4:5
Maintain an attitude of praise and thanksgiving.	Neh. 8:10; Ps. 139:14; Prov. 17:22; Phil. 4:4
Focus on positive emotions, always looking for the good in others and in your life.	Phil. 4:8
Remember to treat your body as the dwelling place of the Holy Spirit.	Rom. 12:1,2; I Cor. 6:19, 20; I Cor. 10:31
Do that which is right and good in the sight of the Lord.	Deut. 6:18

NOTES AND REFERENCES

Chapter 1

1 Recent CT scans dispute this theory.
2 Covington, Richard: *King Tut*, <u>Smithsonian</u>, June 2005, p. 106
3 See Oakes L and Gahlin, L, *Ancient Egypt*, p. 114, 115.
4 This can be a bit confusing at first. One must remember that the geography of Egypt is expressed in relation to the 6,400 kilometer (4000 mile) Nile River which has its headwaters in Central Africa. The Nile, the world's longest river, empties into the Mediterranean Sea through a wide delta. Since the delta is lower in elevation than the more mountainous regions of southern Egypt, northern Egypt is known as lower Egypt while the southern part of the country is referred to as upper Egypt.
5 National Geographic Society video program. *Egypt: Secrets of the Pharaohs*, 1997.
6 For more details see, Ghaliongui, Paul. *The House of Life: Magic and Medical Science in Ancient Egypt*, p. 31–37.
7 Ghaliongui, Paul, *The House of Life*, p. 40.
8 Thorwald, J, *Science and Secrets of Early Medicine*, p. 60.
9 Ghaliongui, Paul, *The House of Life*, p. 44.
10 White, E. G., *The New Illustrated Great Controversy*.
11 Thorwald, J. *op. cit.*, p. 26
12 *Ibid*, p. 27.
13 Bettmann, Otto L, *A Pictorial History of Medicine*, p. 2.
14 *Ibid*, p. 5.
15 *Seventh-day Adventist Bible Commentary*, *Vol. I*, p. 90–94.
16 Covington, *op. cit.*, p. 106.
17 White, Ellen G, *Patriarchs and Prophets*, p. 471–478

Chapter 2

1 Thorwald, J, *Science and Secrets of Early Medicine*, p. 41.
2 *Ibid*, p. 43.
3 Bettmann, O., *A Pictorial History of Medicine*, p. 13.
4 Hanlon, John J, *Public Health Administration and Practice*, p. 14.

5 Psalms 78:25.
6 Psalms 105:40.
7 Joshua 5:11, 12.
8 Bettmann, O., p. 13.
9 White, E. G., *Counsels on Diet and Foods*, p. 378.

Chapter 3

1 Swinson, Arthur, *The History of Public Health*, p. 19.
2 Bettmann, Otto, *A Pictorial History of Medicine*, p. 30.
3 Ackernecht, Edwin H, *A Short History of Medicine*, p. 90.
4 Haggard, Howard, *The Doctor in History*, p. 174.
5 Hubbard, Reuben A, *Historical Perspectives of Religion and Health*, p. 144.
6 Ackernecht, *op. cit.* p. 89.
7 Gordon, Benjamin Lee, *Medieval and Renaissance Medicine*, p. 428.
8 *Ibid.*
9 Haggard, *op. cit.* p. 136.
10 Bettmann, *op. cit.* p. 68.
11 Hubbard, *op. cit.* p. 154.
12 *Ibid.*

Chapter 4

1 For an account of many stories of early Adventists see John Loughborough's *The Great Second Advent Movement*.
2 White, E. G., *Life Sketches*, p. 165, 166.
3 White, E. G., *Life Sketches*, p. 165, 166.
4 *Ibid*, p. 147.
5 White, E. G., *The Ministry of Healing*, p. 17.
6 National Center for Health Statistics (2003).
7 Schaefer, Richard A., *Legacy*, p. 83.
8 National Vital Statistics Reports, Vol. 54, No. 14, April 19, 2006, p. 34. Accessed at http://www.cdc.gov/nchs/fastasts/lifexpec.htm.
9 Schaefer, Richard A., *Legacy*, p. 83.
10 National Vital Statistics Reports, Vol. 54, No. 14, April 19, 2006, p. 35. Accessed at http://www.cdc.gov/nchs/fastats/lifexpec.htm.
11 Rothstein, W. G., *American Physicians in the 19th Century*, p. 56.
12 White, E. G., *Life Sketches*, p. 256.
13 White, E. G., *II Selected Messages*, p. 464.

14 White, E. G., *The Ministry of Healing*, p. 274.
15 Quoted in Rothstein, W. G., *op. cit.* p. 267.
16 *Ibid*, p. 58.
17 *Ibid*, p. 58, 59.
18 White, E. G., *Life Sketches*, p. 137.
19 Rothstein, W. G., *op. cit.* p. 59.
20 White, E. G., *op. cit.* p. 145.
21 Rothstein, *op. cit.* p. 47–49.
22 Dr. Zebra. *President George Washington: Medical History.* Accessed at http://www.doctorzebra.com/prez/g01.htm.
23 *Ibid.*
24 Bettmann, Otto, *A Pictorial History of Medicine*, p. 225.
25 Cited by Rothstein, *op. cit.* p. 191.
26 Hooker, Worthington. *Rational Therapeutics.* Boston: John Wilson and Sons, 1857, p. 40.
27 White, E. G., *Spiritual Gifts, Vol. 4*, p. 138–140.
28 Schaeffer, R. A., op. cit., p. 78–80.
29 Holmes, Oliver Wendall: *Medical Essays, 1842–1882.* Cited in Rothstein, WG: *American Physicians in the 19th Century*, p. 178.
30 Goodwin, Doris Kearns. *Team of Rivals.* New York: Simon and Schuster, 2005, p. 42, 43.
31 Sims J Marion, *The Story of My Life*, p. 150. Cited in Rothstein, WG, *American Physicians in the 19th Century*, p. 62.

Chapter 5

1 Cited in Beller, Susan P., *Medical Practices in the Civil War, p. 19.*
2 *Ibid*, p. 24.
3 Fowler, Robert H., *Gettysburg*, p. 61.
4 For a full account of the story see, Coon, Roger G. *The Great Visions of Ellen White*, chapter 7.
5 White, Ellen G., *Spiritual Gifts, Vol. 4*, p. 148.
6 *Ibid*, p. 134
7 *Ibid*, p. 126
8 *Ibid*, p. 128
9 *Ibid*, p. 139
10 *Ibid*, p. 120
11 *Ibid.*
12 *Ibid*, p. 145
13 *Ibid*, p. 134, 136.
14 *Ibid*, p. 140

15 *Ibid*, p. 141
16 White, Ellen G., *Manuscript 1*, 1863, p. 6
17 James Nix presentation at Adventist Heritage Village, Battle Creek, MI during 2006 local ASI convention.
18 Kellogg, John Harvey, Preface to *Christian Temperance and Bible Hygiene*, p. iii.
19 *Ibid.*
20 Franklin, Benjamin, *The Autobiography of Benjamin Franklin*, p. 88, 89.
21 Cayleff, Susan E., In *Other Healers: Unorthodox Medicine in America*, p. 83.
22 White, Ellen G., *Life Sketches*, p. 168–170 and *Testimonies to the Church, Vol. 1*, p. 615–618.
23 White, Ellen G., *Second Advent Review and Sabbath Herald*, October 8, 1867.
24 Loughborough, J. N., *The Great Second Advent Movement*, p. 364, 365.

Chapter 6

1 White, Ellen G., *Christ's Object Lessons*, p. 327.
2 White, Ellen G., *Testimonies for the Church Vol. 1*, p. 486 and *Testimonies for the Church Vol. 7*, p. 59.
3 White, Ellen G., *Life Sketches*, p. 169.
4 White, Ellen G., *Testimonies for the Church, Vol. 1*, p. 615.
5 Kellogg, Merritt G., *A Bit of Family History*, July 6, 1914.
6 *Ibid.*
7 *Ibid.*
8 As told by Schaeffer, Richard A., *Legacy, p. 125.*
9 White, Ellen G., *Selected Messages Vol. II*, p. 211.
10 Schaeffer, Richard, *Legacy*, p. 128.
11 Kellogg, John Harvey, *Biographical Facts*, June 13, 1940.
12 Wiggam, Albert Edward, *American Magazine*, Dec. 1925.
13 *Ibid.*
14 Kellogg, John Harvey, *op. cit.*, 1940.
15 Schwarz, Richard W., *John Harvey Kellogg, M.D.*, p. 113.
16 Kellogg, John Harvey, *op. cit.*, 1940.
17 White, Ellen G., Reprinted in *Battle Creek Letters*. Letter to Dr. Kellogg dated January 12, 1900.
18 Quoted by Schaeffer, Richard in *Legacy*, p. 137.
19 Schwartz, Richard W., *John Harvey Kellogg, M.D.*, p. 133.
20 Jemison, T. H., *A Prophet Among You*, p. 491, 492.

Chapter 7

1 *Titanic* — http://www.keyflux.com/titanic/facts.htm

2 Bill Hughes in *The Secret Terrorists*, provides a plausible but stunning possibility. See pages 57–63.

3 Mowbray, J. H., *The Sinking of the Titanic*, 1912. http://gaslight.mtroyal.ab.ca/titanic.htm Accessed on March 18, 2006.

4 White, Ellen G., *Selected Messages*, Vol. 1, p. 205, 206.

5 Mowbray, J. H., *The Sinking of the Titanic*.

6 White, Ellen G., *Selected Messages*, Vol. 1, p. 200.

7 Hook, Milton, *Flames Over Battle Creek*, p. 98.

8 Walton, Lewis, *Omega*, p.12 and *Omega II*, p. 10.

9 Walton, Lewis, *Omega II*, p. 14.

10 White, Ellen G., *Letter 3, 1900*.

11 White, Ellen G., *Letter K – 204 — 99*, reprinted in *Battle Creek Letters*.

12 White, Ellen G., *Letter K – 215 — 99*, reprinted in *Battle Creek Letters*.

13 *Movement of Destiny* is the name Elder LeRoy Froom gave to his book on the history of Adventism.

14 Gerstner, Patsy in *The Temple of Health. A Pictorial History of the Battle Creek Sanitarium, p. 25*

15 White, Ellen G., *Letter B — 128 — 02*, reprinted in *Battle Creek Letters*.

16 Kellogg, John H., Preface to *Christian Temperance and Bible Hygiene*.

17 White, Ellen G., *Testimonies for the Church*, Vol. 8, p. 291.

18 White, Ellen G. Letter 179, 1904. Quoted in *Counsels to Writers and Editors*, p. 93.

19 Walton, Lewis, *Omega II*, p. 35, 36.

20 White, Ellen G., *Testimonies for the Church*, vol. 8, p. 97.

21 Cited by Gerstner, Patsy, *op. cit, p. 31*.

22 The New Temple of Health, *Battle Creek Idea*, May, 1904, 1–2.

23 Schaefer, Richard A., *Legacy*, p. 128–130.

24 *Battle Creek Daily News*. Worst conflagration ever visited on our city. February 18, 1902.

25 Schwartz, Richard W., *John Harvey Kellogg, M.D.*, p. 188.

26 Kellogg interview with A. C. Bordeau and A. G. Amandon, October 7, 1907.

27 *Ibid*

28 Office of Public Affairs. *The Hart-Dole-Inouye Federal Center: A Historic Guide*, p. 14–17.

29 *Ibid*, p 16.
30 *Ibid*.
31 White, Ellen G., *Testimonies for the Church, Vol. 8*, p. 105, 106.
32 http://www.adventist.ord/world_church/facts_and_figures/index.html Accessed on March 19, 2006
33 Walton, Lewis R., *Omega II*, p. 199, 200.
34 *Ibid*, p. 199

Chapter 8

1 White, Ellen G., *Letter B — 128 — 02* written July 6, 1902. Cited in *Battle Creek Letters*, p. 50.
2 White, Ellen G., *Testimonies for the Church*, vol. 9, p. 173.
3 Cited by Schaeffer, Richard A., in *Legacy*, p. 171, 172. Taken from a letter from John A. Burden to E. H. Risley, M.D., dated June 3, 1929.
4 Schaeffer, Richard A, *Legacy*, p. 171,172.
5 White, Ellen G., *Testimonies for the Church, Vol. 9*, p. 271, 272.

Chapter 9

1 Wnyder, Ernst, et al., *Cancer Research*, December 1953.
2 Lemon, Frank R., et al., *Cancer*, 1964.
3 Adventist Health Study, http://www.llu.edu/llu health/abstracts/
4 Philips, Roland L, *Journal of Environmental Pathology and Toxicology*, 1980 and Philips, Roland L. et al., *J. National Cancer Inst.* 1980.
5 Lemon, Frank R. and Kuzma, Jan W, *Archives of Environmental Health*, 1969.
6 Philips, Roland L., et al., *American Journal of Clinical Nutrition*, 1978.
7 World Health Organization, http://3.who.int/whosis/mort/table1_process.cfm
8 Philips, Roland L, et al., *American Journal of Clinical Nutrition*, 1978 and Marmot, M. G., et al., *American J. of Epidemiology*, 1975.
9 Waaler, H and Hjort, P. F., *Journal of the Norwegian Medical Association*, 1981.
10 Ibid.
11 Hirayama, T, *British Medical Journal*, 1981.
12 Hirayama T, *National Cancer Institute Monographs*, 1985.

206 • Adventist Heritage of Health

13 Personal conversation with Dr. Charles Thomas, Ph.D, former instructor at Loma Linda University, School of Public Health.
14 Hubbard J D; Inkeles S; Barnard R J: Nathan Pritikin's Heart. *New England Journal of Medicine*, July 4, *1985*.
15 White, Ellen G., *Counsels on Diet and Foods*, p. 414, 415.

Chapter 10

1 Canfield, Jack and Hansen, Mark V. "Who You Are Makes a Difference" in *Chicken Soup for the Soul*. Deerfield Beach, FL: Health Communications, Inc., pp. 19–21 as submitted by Helice Bridges.

Chapter 11

1 Cited by Coon, Roger W. in *The Great Visions of Ellen G. White*, p. 105.
2 White, Ellen G., *Counsels on Diet and Foods*, p. 377.
3 White, Ellen G., *Christian Temperance and Bible Hygiene*, p. 53.

Chapter 12

1 Malkmus, George, *How to Eliminate Sickness*. Video presentation. Hallelujah Acres, Shelby, NC, 1987.
2 *National Geographic Magazine*, November 2005.
3 Joshua 8:33–35.
4 Psalms 103:3
5 Isaiah 40:31

BIBLIOGRAPHY
of Major Works Cited

Chapters 1, 2

Ackerknecht, Edwin H. *A Short History of Medicine*. Baltimore, MD: John Hopkins University Press, 1982.

Bettmann, Otto L. *A Pictorial History of Medicine*. Springfield, IL: Charles C. Thomas Publisher, 1979.

Ghaliougui, Paul. *The House of Life – Magic and Medical Science in Ancient Egypt*. Amsterdam, Netherlands: B.M. Israel, 1963.

Hubbard, Reuben A. *Historical Perspectives of Religion and Health*. Berrien Springs, MI: Andrews University, 1986.

Nunn, John F. *Ancient Egyptian Medicine*. Norman, OK: University of Oklahoma Press, 1996.

Oakes, Lorna and Gahlin, Lucia. *Ancient Egypt*. New York: Hermes House, 2002.

Thorwald, Jurgen. *Science and Secrets of Early Medicine*. New York, NY: Harcourt, Brace, and World, 1962.

Chapter 3

Ackerknecht, Edwin H. *A Short History of Medicine*. Baltimore, MD: John Hopkins University Press, 1982.

Bettmann, Otto L. *A Pictorial History of Medicine*. Springfield, IL: Charles C. Thomas Publisher, 1979.

EyeWitness to History. "Black Death, 1348," www.eyewitnesstohistory.com (2001).

Halsall, Paul. Edward Grim: The Murder of Thomas Becket. *Internet Medieval Source Book*. Accessed at www. fordham.edu/halsall/source/grim-becket.html.

Hubbard, Reuben A. *Historical Perspectives of Religion and Health*. Berrien Springs, MI: Andrews University, 1986.

Chapter 4

Dr. Zebra. *President George Washington: Medical History*. Accessed at http://www.doctorzebra.com/prez/g01.htm

Loughborough, J. N. *The Great Second Advent Movement*. Southern Publishing Assoc., 1905. Reprinted by Adventist Pioneer Library, 1992.

Rothstein, William G. *American Physicians in the 19th Century*. Baltimore, MD: John Hopkins University Press, 1972.

Schaefer, Richard A. *Legacy*. Loma Linda, CA: Legacy Publishing Assoc., 1990.

White, Ellen G. *Life Sketches*. Mountain View, CA: Pacific Press Pub. Assn., 1915.

White, Ellen G. *Selected Messages, Vol 2*. Washington D.C.: Review and Herald Publishing Assoc.,1958.

White, Ellen G. *Spiritual Gifts, Vol. IV*. Washington D.C.: Review and Herald Publishing Assoc.

Chapter 5

Beller, Susan P. *Medical Practices in the Civil War*. Charlotte, VT: Self-published, 1992.

Coon, Roger W. *The Great Visions of Ellen White*. Hagerstown, MD: Review and Herald Pub. Assn., 1992.

Fowler, Robert H., editor. *Gettysburg*. Gettysburg, PA: Historical Times Inc., 1963.

Gevitz, Norman, ed. *Other Healers: Unorthodox Medicine in America,Balimore*, MD: The Johns Hopkins University Press, 1988.

White, Ellen G. *Selected Messages, Vol 2*. Washington D.C.: Review and Herald Publishing Assoc.,1958.

White, Ellen G. *Spiritual Gifts, Vol. IV.* Washington D.C.: Review and Herald Publishing Assoc.

Whorton, James C. *Nature Cures – The History of Alternative Medicine in America*. New York, NY: Oxford University Press, 2002.

Chapter 6

Jemison, T. Housel. *A Prophet Among You*. Mountain View, CA: Pacific Press Pub. Assn., 1955.

Kellogg, John Harvey (June 13, 1940). *Biographical Facts.* Folder "Autobiographical/ Biographical," John Harvey Kellogg Papers 1832–1943, Box 1, Bentley Historical Library, University of Michigan.

Kellogg, Merritt G (1914) *A Bit of Family History – July 6, 1914.* Folder "Autobiographical/ Biographical," John Harvey Kellogg Collection, Box 1, Bentley Historical Library, University of Michigan.

Schaefer, Richard A. *Legacy.* Loma Linda, CA: Legacy Publishing Assoc., 1990.

Schwarz, Richard W. *John Harvey Kellogg, M.D.* Nashville, TN: Southern Publishing Assoc., 1970.

White, Ellen G. *Battle Creek Letters*. Payson, AZ: Leaves of Autumn Books, 1999.

Wiggam, Albert Edward. The most remarkable man I have ever known. *American Magazine*, Dec. 1925, p. 14–15, 117–118.

Chapter 7

Gertsner, Patsy. *The Temple of Health. A Pictorial History of the Battle Creek Sanitarium.* Southern Illinois University, 1996.

Kellogg, John Harvey. October 7th 1907 interview with Elders A. C. Bordeau and G. W. Amadon. Accessed at http://www.ex-sda.com/john.htm.

Mowbray, JH. *The Sinking of the Titanic,* 1912. Accessed at http://gaslight.mtroyal.ab.ca/titanic.htm.

Office of Public Affairs. The Hart-Dole-Inouye Federal Center: *A Historic Guide,* Battle Creek, MI, 2004.

Schwarz, Richard W. *John Harvey Kellogg, M.D.* Nashville, TN: Southern Publishing Assoc., 1970.

Titanic — http://www.keyflux.com/titanic/facts.htm. Accessed on March 18, 2006.

Walton, Lewis R. *Omega. Washington D.C.: Review and Herald Publishing Assoc.,1981.*

Walton, Lewis R. *Omega II.* Glennville, CA: Lewis R. Walton, 1995.

White, Ellen G. *Battle Creek Letters.* Payson, AZ: Leaves of Autumn Books, 1999.

White, Ellen G. *Testimonies to the Church, Vol. 8.* Mountain View, CA: Pacific Press Publishing Assoc., 1948.

Chapter 8

Schaefer, Richard A. *Legacy.* Loma Linda, CA: Legacy Publishing Assoc., 1990.

Chapter 9

Nelson, Ethel R. *Eight Secrets of Health.* Bangkok, Thailand: Thailand Publishing House, 1991.

Adventist Health Study. *Bibliography of Health-related Research Studies among Seventh-day Adventists*. Accessed at http://www.llu.edu/llu/health/abstracts/

Chapter 10

Andress, William and Gohde, Winnie. *Grandma Whitney Queen of the Mountain*. Brushton, NY: Teach Services, 1996.

Hardinge, Mervyn G. *My Unexpected Life*. Brushton, NY: Teach Services, 2005.

Moore, Raymond S. *China Doctor*. Mountain View, CA: Pacific Press Pub. Assn., 1969.

Other References Cited in Alphabetical Order by Author

Brosco, Jeffrey P. The early history of the infant mortality rate in America: "A reflection upon the past and a prophecy of the future" *Pediatrics* Vol. 103 No. 2, February 1999, pp. 478–485.

Buettner, Dan: The secrets of living longer. *National Geographic Magazine*, p. 2–27, November 2005.

Franklin, Benjamin. *Autobiography of Benjamin Franklin, The 2nd edition*. New Haven, CT: Yale University Press, 2003.

Goodwin, Doris Kearns. *Team of Rivals*. New York: Simon and Schuster, 2005.

Gordon, Benjamin Lee. *Medieval and Renaissance Medicine*, New York: Philosophical Library, 1959.

Haggard, Howard W. *The Doctor in History*. New Haven: Yale University Press, 1934.

Hanlon, John J. *Public Health Administration and Practice*. St. Louis, MO: C.V. Mosby Co., 1979.

Hirayama, T: Non-smoking wives of heavy smokers have a higher risk of lung cancer: a study from Japan. *British Medical Journal* 282:183–85, Jan. 1981.

Hirayama T: Mortality in Japanese with lifestyles similar to Seventh-day Adventists: a strategy for risk reduction by life-style modification. *National Cancer Institute Monographs* 1985;69:143–53.

Hook, Milton. *Flames Over Battle Creek*. Washington D.C.: Review and Herald Publishing Assoc., 1977.

Hughes, Bill. *The Secret Terrorists*. Tangerine, FL: Truth Triumphant, 2002.

Leake, Chauncy D. *The Old Egyptian Medical Papyri*. Lawrence, KS: University of Kansas Press, 1952.

Lemon, Frank R, Walden, Richard T, and Woods, Robert W: Cancer of the lung and mouth in Seventh-day Adventists. *Cancer* 17:486–497, 1964.

Lemon, Frank R. and Kuzma, Jan W: Biologic cost of smoking: Decreased life expectancy. *Archives of Environmental Health* 18:950–955, 1969.

Marmot, MG, Syme SL, Kagan A, et.al: Epidemiologic studies of coronary heart disease and stroke in Japanese men living in Japan, Hawaii, and California. *American J. of Epidemiology* 102:514–524, 1975.

National Geographic Society video program. *Egypt: Secrets of the Pharaohs*. Washington D.C., 1997.

Philips RL., Lemon FR, Beeson WL, and Kuzma JW: Coronary heart disease mortality among Seventh-day Adventists with differing dietary habits: a preliminary report. *American Journal of Clinical Nutrition* 31:S191–S198, 1978.

Philips, Roland L: Cancer among Seventh-day Adventists. *Journal of Environmental Pathology and Toxicology* 3:157–169, 1980.

Philips, RL, Garfinkel L, Kuzma JW, Beeson WL, Lotz TL, and Brin B: Mortality among California Seventh-day Adventists for selected cancer sites. *J. National Cancer Inst.* 65(5):1097–1107, November 1980.

Seventh-day Adventist Church. *Seventh-day Adventist World Church Statistics*. http://www.adventist.org/world_church/facts_and_figures/index.html.

Seventh-day Adventist Bible Commentary, Vol. 1. Hagerstown, MD: Review and Herald Publishing Assoc., 1978.

Swinson, Arthur. *The History of Public Health*. Exeter, Wheaton, 1966.

Waaler, H and Hjort, PF: Low mortality among Norwegian Seventh-day Adventists 1960–1977: A message on lifestyle and health? *Journal of the Norwegian Medical Association* 101(11): 623–627, 1981.

White, Ellen G and James S. *Christian Temperance and Bible Hygiene*. Battle Creek, MI: Good Health Publishing Co, 1890. Reprinted by Leaves of Autumn Books in 1980.

White, Ellen G. *Christ's Object Lessons*. Washington D.C.: Review and Herald Publishing Assoc.,1941.

White, Ellen G. *Counsels on Diet and Foods*. Takoma Park, MD: Review and Herald Publishing Assoc.,1946.

White, Ellen G. *Counsels to Writers and Editors*. Nashville, TN: Southern Publishing Assoc., 1946.

White, Ellen G. *Desire of Ages, The*. Mountain View, CA, Pacific Press Publishing Assoc. 1940.

White, Ellen G. *The Ministry of Healing*. Mountain View, CA, Pacific Press Publishing Assoc. 1942.

White, Ellen G. *New Illustrated Great Controversy, The*. Deland, FL: Laymen for Religious Liberty, Inc., 1990

White, Ellen G. *Patriarchs and Prophets*. Mountain View, CA, Pacific Press Pub. Assoc. 1958.

White, Ellen G: *Second Advent Review and Sabbath Herald*, October 8, 1867

White, Ellen G. *Testimonies to the Church, Vol. 1.* Mountain View, CA, Pacific Press Publishing Assoc. 1948.

White, Ellen G. *Testimonies to the Church, Vol. 1.* Mountain View, CA, Pacific Press Publishing Assoc. 1948.

White, Ellen G. *Testimonies to the Church, Vol. 7.* Mountain View, CA, Pacific Press Publishing Assoc. 1948.

White, Ellen G. *Testimonies to the Church, Vol. 9.* Mountain View, CA, Pacific Press Publishing Assoc. 1948.

Wnyder, Ernst et.al: Experimental production of carcinoma with tobacco tar. *Cancer Research* 13:855–864, December 1953.

World Health Organization. http://www3.who.int/whosis/mort/table1_process.cfm.

SCRIPTURAL INDEX

215

We'd love to have you download our catalog of
titles we publish at:

www.TEACHServices.com

or write or email us your thoughts,
reactions, or criticism about this
or any other book we publish at:

TEACH Services, Inc.
254 Donovan Road
Brushton, NY 12916

info@TEACHServices.com

or you may call us at:

518/358-3494